# Movement Difficulties in Developmental Disorders

# Movement Difficulties in Developmental Disorders

## Practical Guidelines for Assessment and Management

**David Sugden**

Emeritus Professor, School of Education,
University of Leeds, Leeds, UK

**Michael G Wade**

Professor, Motor Learning/Motor Development, School of Kinesiology,
University of Minnesota, Minneapolis, USA

2019
Mac Keith Press

© 2019 Mac Keith Press

Managing Director: Ann-Marie Halligan
Senior Publishing Manager: Sally Wilkinson
Publishing Co-ordinator: Lucy White
Project Management: Riverside Publishing Solutions Ltd

The views and opinions expressed herein are those of the authors and do not necessarily represent those of the publisher.

First published in this edition in 2019 by Mac Keith Press
2nd Floor, Rankin Building, 139–143 Bermondsey Street, London, SE1 3UW

British Library Cataloguing-in-Publication data
A catalogue record for this book is available from the British Library

Cover designer: Hannah Rogers

ISBN: 978-1-909962-94-1

Typeset by Riverside Publishing Solutions Ltd

Printed by Hobbs the Printers Ltd, Totton, Hampshire, UK

# Dedication

In the final stages of this book David Sugden became increasingly incapacitated as a result of a courageous, four year struggle, with cancer. David died March 13th 2019 and this book, among his many other contributions, represents his ongoing commitment to both academic research and the clinical applications, that research affords all professionals and parents, who daily seek to improve the lives of special needs children.

# Contents

# Notable Clinicians Appointments

**Professor Anna Barnett**
Professor of Psychology, Department of Psychology, Health and Professional Development, Oxford Brookes University, Oxford, UK

**Professor Reint H Geuze**
Emeritus Associate Professor, Faculty of Behavioural and Social Sciences, University of Groningen, Groningen, The Netherlands

**Professor Beth Hands**
Professor, Senior Research Scholar, Institute for Health Research, The University of Notre Dame, Fremantle, Australia

**Professor Sheila E Henderson**
Chair of the Friends of Sawbridgeworth Neuro Centres; Emeritus Professor of Developmental Psychology, Department of Psychology and Human Development, UCL Institute of Education, University College London, London, UK

**Professor Amanda Kirby**
CEO of Do IT Solutions Ltd; Chair, Developmental Disorders in Education, University of South Wales, Wales, UK

**Dr Victoria McQuillan**
Lecturer in Occupational Therapy, School of Health Sciences, The University of Liverpool, Liverpool, UK

**Professor Cheryl Missiuna**
Professor, School of Rehabilitation Science; John & Margaret Lillie Chair in Childhood Disability Research; Scientist and Past Director, CanChild, McMaster University, Hamilton, Canada

**Dr Motohide Myahara**
Associate Professor, School of Physical Education, Sport and Exercise Sciences, University of Otago, New Zealand and Visiting Research Fellow, Department of Neuropsychiatry, School of Medicine, Hirosaki University, Aomori, Japan

**Professor Helene Polatajko**
Professor, Department of Occupational Science and Occupational Therapy, University of Toronto, Toronto, Canada

**Dr Mellissa Prunty**
Senior Lecturer in Occupational Therapy, Brunel University, London, UK

**Dr Marina M Schoemaker**
Associate Professor, University of Groningen, University Medical Centre, Centre of Human Movement Science, Groningen, the Netherlands

**Professor Bouwien Smits-Engelsman**
Professor in Developmental Human movement Science, University of Cape Town, South Africa

**Professor Peter Wilson**
Professor of Developmental Psychology; Co-Director, Centre for Disability & Development Research (CeDDR), School of Behavioural and Health Science, Faculty of Health Sciences, Australian Catholic University, Melbourne, Australia

# Foreword

In the 1980's, I was asked to review a book by Jack Keogh and David Sugden on motor skill development. I loved their book (Keogh & Sugden, 1985). They had written a text that offered a unique and important perspective on the field of motor development. And now in 2019, I once again find myself loving a book by David Sugden – this time with co-author Michael Wade. The current book shares with the reader, the wisdom of these two scholars who have spent their careers engaged in the scientific study of motor learning and development, assessment, and intervention to better understand those with movement difficulties. With this book, they have found a way to communicate their vast knowledge in an accessible and relevant manner for those working with individuals with developmental disorders who have movement disorders.

The book starts by laying out the authors 'triad' of influences on movement outcomes. In their triad model, an individual's motor behavior and subsequent development emerges from that individual's resources (e.g. strength, perceptual abilities), the environmental context in which that individual functions (e.g. home, community), and the task at hand (e.g. spoon use, catching a ball). This triad is woven throughout the book as the authors present theoretical, empirical, and professional evidence to support parents, teachers, therapists and others who work with individuals who have movement difficulties.

From the theory and research, Sugden and Wade present useful guidance and support on assessment and intervention. Intertwined throughout the book are case studies that move from the general account of assessment and intervention to practical, real life situations.Interspersed in each chapter are summary boxes that highlight important principles, definitions, and resources. Case studies are also strategically placed to bring out key ideas that are intended to emphasize and explain the principles presented.

For those who want to understand more deeply how motor skills are learned, the authors offer an excellent and readable summary of motor learning principles in chapter two. Examples of how these principles would inform practice and instruction are provided. The practitioners and clinicians should find the information accessible and related to their challenges in working with those who have movement difficulties. These principles are a recurring theme throughout the remaining chapters on objectives to action and specific guidelines for intervention.

A unique contribution of the book is the chapter that includes interviews with prominent clinicians and researchers in the field of movement difficulties. These thirteen internationally well-known authorities offer their unique, tested, and well-thought out ideas on intervention strategies and guidelines for those with movement difficulties. As the authors argue and I agree, who better to provide evidence and insights to inform best practices than this group of individuals.

Overall, if you are someone who works with those with developmental disorders and who have movement difficulties, this is a book you want to read and re-read. In a year, your copy of the book should be well worn as you visit and re-visit the abundance of ideas that Sugden and Wade offer in this book.

Finally, I cannot close this Foreword without expressing my deep sadness at the passing of David Sugden in March 2019. We can all be thankful that he completed this book before his untimely death, but, at least for me, I will greatly miss reading a new Sugden book.

## Reference

Keogh J, Sugden DA (1985) *Movement skill development*. New York: Macmillan.

**Jane E. Clark**
Professor Emerita
Department of Kinesiology, School of Public Health
University of Maryland

# Preface

This text is aimed at those professionals, parents and others who work with children showing movement difficulties. The core of the text is focused on children with what is now called Developmental Coordination Disorder (DCD), the international term for what is often called dyspraxia. It is also aimed at those individuals who show movement difficulties as a *secondary* and co-occurring characteristic such as children on the autistic spectrum (ASD), those with generic learning difficulties such as dyslexia, attention deficit disorder and speech and language impairment. Children with cerebral palsy (CP) were not specifically included as this condition is typically a special case with specific medical assessments and intervention options, sometimes surgical. To include these would alter the nature of the text, although we do recognize that some of the principles and methods in this book will apply to children with CP. The book does not adopt any particular *'method'*, although it obviously touches upon various approaches that are currently available. The emphasis is on exploiting the principles and practices sign posted by evidence-based research, informed by extant theory, empirical evidence and professional expertise.

We have attempted to bring together evidence-based knowledge from research and how that knowledge can be integrated into both assessment, diagnosis and clinical intervention that seeks optimize positive outcomes for children with movement difficulties. The early chapters cover both the nature of the difficulties experienced by children, the underlying principles of motor learning that might account for the movement difficulties and how assessment and diagnosis might be achieved. The chapters following address description, assigned labels and terminology. The latter part of the book engage the specific actions and guidelines to address the range of movement difficulties of children with a range of specific deficits, with respect to their movement repertoire. We close the book with a series of interviews from well-known academics and clinicians who provide useful insights into the role and impact of the different methodologies discussed and reviewed in the book.

**Michael Wade**

# Chapter 1

# The nature of movement difficulties and developmental disorders

## Movement

Movement is a core characteristic of all humans and is an essential part of our every-day existence. One has only to think of what we do from getting up in the morning to retiring in the evening to recognize just how fundamental movement is to our daily living. One can go further and say that movement is the only facility we have that allows us to interact with both other humans and our environment (Wolpert et al. 2003). Movement is not only important in its own right, but also supports other faculties, such as language, cognition and social interaction. This has often been referred to as 'embod-ied cognition' (Smith and Gasser 2005; Bornstein et al. 2013). In their seminal work *Travel Broadens the Mind*, Joe Campos and colleagues (2000) carefully illustrate the way 'travel', that is, locomotion in infancy, is a spur to the development of other attributes, including language, attention and cognition, as well as personality characteristics such as resilience. It is linked to deep-seated sets of changes in perception, spatial cognition and social development. Locomotion in infancy has a transactional function with these other attributes, each one having a bidirectional effect. Thus locomotion in infancy affects and is affected by the faculties of, for example, cognition and social, perceptual and emotional competencies. This concept has been further elaborated by the work on 'embodied cognition' that stresses the strong relationship between cognition and action. As we have noted in other work, the development of action enables the advancement of behavioural flexibility and embodied cognition epitomizes this concept (Sugden and Wade 2013). Thus, movement is a crucial part of our lives, not only in its own right, but also in its contribution to other abilities.

As we watch children develop we chronicle the changes taking place. In infancy these are raising of the head, turning over, reaching and grasping, standing and, of course, the major milestone of walking that occurs around the time of the first birthday. In early childhood, we see children running, jumping, hopping, skipping, catching, writing and drawing and developing many other skills that are part of our daily lives. Most children achieve these skills within a time frame that we would class as typical. There may be delay in some children, but, in general, the majority achieve these milestones with little effort or thought; they occur naturally with maturation and experience.

## How do we view development and learning?

An important feature of motor development and learning is that the same variables or constraints apply to this process in all children, whether their development is typical or atypical. Throughout this text we emphasize that movement development is a function of a triad involving (1) the resources **the child possesses**, (2) the **environment in which the individual functions,** and (3) the **tasks that are presented and manner of the presentation**. These variables or constraints are analysed and described by Newell (1986). The variables are the same in every individual; it is simply the metrics within them constraints that differ. The resources the individual possesses would include not only their movement capabilities, but also their social, emotional and cognitive characteristics. Other attributes important for intervention outcomes, such as resilience and motivation, would also be included here.

The individual's environment is another feature of this triad of parameters. In this context, the questions that need to be considered are, Where does the individual go to school? What are the school practices? What contribution does health and the community make? How does the family fit into this and how can carers/parents be empowered? What are policies at local and national level?

Finally, when the child is in a learning context, how is the learning organized and what tasks are presented and in what manner? How is practice structured both formally and informally? The main and crucially important point of this triad, which is central to this book, is to show that the individual is not the sole unit of analysis in the assessment of his or her movement. It is rather the individual in a specific context, with all the accompanying variables or constraints.

A child with movement difficulties develops and learns within these constraints and in this way, is similar to a child with no difficulties. The differences are the metrics within the constraints. For example, the metrics of the child's resources for movement could include strength, with a child with movement difficulties being weaker than his or her peers. Also, the task could be ideally suited to the child with appropriate instruction,

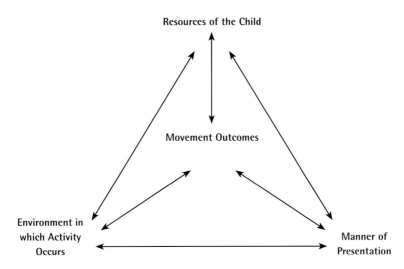

**Figure 1.1** Triad of influences on movement outcomes.

or it may not be suitable. The environment, such as educational and health resources, could be helpful and present or absent; the child him- or herself will have a different set of resources. But fundamentally, these three constraints (the child, the task and the environment) act upon the learning and development of the child and it is these dynamic transactions that are the cornerstones of our approach. This dynamical view of development and learning is at the core of this text that stresses how these ongoing transactions provide the final outcome in development; learning and by association, support and intervention, for those with movement difficulties. This differs greatly from maturational or other theoretical positions, such as information processing, that assert, either directly or tacitly, that the most problems reside solely in the child. Thus, in our approach, the dynamic interaction between the **child**, the **environment** and the **task** is the unit of analysis (see Fig. 1.1).

A simple example of how the task influences action illustrates this point. In a hand reaching and grasping study by Newell et al. (1989) infants reached for an object with one or two hands, according to the size of the object. There was a scaled relationship between the object and the hand-width aperture formed by the thumb and index finger. (We will illustrate this concept in later chapters.) Both development and learning are non-linear, i.e. they do not follow easily prescribed pathways but differ according to the three constraints listed above. Thus, our approach to support for a child learning a skill are also non-linear and are described in detail in Chapters 6 and 7. Suffice to say here that non-linear refers to different progressions among children and different outcomes and is not geared towards fixed methodologies with predetermined objectives. Our approach is to view a situation and flexibly allocate the resources to the demands of that situation by providing functional solutions.

In Chapters 4 and 6 on assessment and intervention we discuss how the triad of child resources, task and context, either general or specific, influence therapy and teaching, no matter the child's ability.

We would add here that while this book focuses on movement, this triad also applies to other aspects of development.

## Resources of the child

While most children will learn movement skills in the expected manner, other children have difficulties and are delayed or impaired in their movements. Some children show difficulties in specific areas while others have global problems. With respect to movement difficulties, children can be roughly divided into two groups: those with movement difficulties as the **primary core defining characteristic** and those with movement difficulties as a **secondary co-occurring characteristic**. While this may appear to be a somewhat reductionist approach, it does help in the describing the movements and in planning and enacting intervention (see Box 1.1).

*Children with movement difficulties as the core defining characteristic*
This group of children includes those who have a movement difficulty as the **core and primary part** of their diagnosis. The group we will be looking at in this regard are children who are diagnosed with developmental coordination disorder (DCD). The term dyspraxia is also used to describe these children in the UK but with a slightly different definition. However, we prefer the term DCD that is used internationally by the American Psychiatric Association (APA 2013) and the World Health Organization, and has been the subject of 12 international conferences every 2 years, from the first one

---

**Box 1.1** Primary and secondary movement difficulties

**Children with movement difficulties as a defining characteristic**

✓ Developmental coordination disorder
✓ Cerebral palsy
✓ Other

**Children with movement difficulties as a secondary co-occurring characteristic**

✓ Dyslexia
✓ Developmental language disorder
✓ Attention-deficit–hyperactivity disorder
✓ Autism spectrum disorder
✓ Other

in 1993 in London to the latest in Perth, Australia in 2017. It is also the preferred term of the recent DSM-5 (APA 2103) and recent *International Clinical Practice Guidelines on Definition, Diagnosis, Assessment, Intervention and Psycho-social Aspects of Developmental Coordination Disorder* (Blank et al. 2019). However, this text does not solely concern DCD as this, we believe, would be too narrow, particularly given our focus on addressing the all the symptoms experienced by the child. There will be children with movement difficulties as their primary problem but who do not have a formal diagnosis. Most of the evidence for intervention comes from the population with DCD, because a movement disorder is the defining core characteristic in this condition and these children represent a significant prevalence of around 2% to 6%, depending on definitional and diagnostic markers. However, as we note later, there are some estimates of prevalence that are as high as 15%.

This book is not specifically concerned with children with cerebral palsy, or other known genotypes such as fragile X, Duchenne muscular dystrophy, or Down syndrome, mainly because some of these conditions will have interventions that involve surgery and other specialist techniques and approaches that are beyond the scope of this book. However, many of the general principles and practices pertaining to support described in this book can be applied to these populations in certain circumstances. For example, the triad of variables illustrated in Figure 1.1 is the same for all populations. As we noted earlier, it is the metrics within these variables that differ.

*Children with movement difficulties as a secondary co-occurring characteristic*
The second group of children who show movement difficulties are those whose primary defining characteristics are in the cognitive, social, linguistic, literacy and emotional and behavioural fields, with movement being a **secondary characteristic**. These are children described as having dyslexia (DYX), autism spectrum disorder (ASD), developmental language disorder (DLD), and attention-deficit–hyperactivity disorder (ADHD). While not all of these children will have movement difficulties as part of their profile, as a group they show a higher prevalence of motor disorders than their typically developing, age-matched peers. All of these disorders, including DCD, are categorized as 'neurodevelopmental disorders'. This is a 'coarse-grained' label, but in journals such as *Research in Developmental Disorders* or in university courses in education, psychology or health studies, this term would be recognized as one that has the best fit across these children.

*Details of the children with developmental coordination disorder*
Children with movement difficulties have been described for some time by parents, educators, health professionals and others as being 'clumsy' often with reference to a 'Clumsy Child Syndrome'. The term 'developmental coordination disorder' refers to a condition with movement difficulties being the core of any definition and, thus,

> **Box 1.2** DSM-5 definition of developmental coordination disorder
>
> **There are four criteria specified by DSM-5 (APA 2013) for a diagnosis of DCD:**
>
> A. Coordination is substantially below that expected for chronological age and shown by clumsiness in the execution of skills or slow and inaccurate performance of movement skills. Thus, a selection of activities such as bumping into people or objects, dropping objects, untidy and slow handwriting and poor recreational skills such as in bike ride or ball games are characteristic. Ideally addressing Criterion A would involve a clinical synthesis of:
>
>    ✓ Developmental and medical history
>
>    ✓ School or work place report
>
>    ✓ Individual assessment using psychometrically sound and culturally appropriate standardized tests
>
>    ✓ Care with delay as opposed to deficit, variability in performance and awkward, slow and less precise performance
>
> B. The difficulties in A above interfere and cause problems in the activities of daily living such as in self-care, schoolwork, leisure and recreational activities or work-related problems. In adults, this could involve speed and accuracy on some tasks.
>
> C. The start of the difficulties is in the developmental period. DCD is not typically diagnosed below 5 years of age because of variability in both development and experience. However, non-diagnosis does not mean difficulties should go unnoticed or ignore. Support can be given in a graded fashion as in responses to intervention methods in reading.
>
> D. The problems are not better explained by other disorders such as intellectual difficulties, definable neurological conditions such as cerebral palsy or visual impairment. Visual function and neural examination must be included in diagnostic evaluation. There is no IQ cut off or discrepancy invoked but if intellectual disability is present, motor difficulties are in excess of those expected by mental age. It is worth noting that as IQ dips below 70ish, prevalence of motor difficulties increases exponentially.

movement is viewed as being the primary characteristic. Box 1.2 shows the latest definition of DCD as contained in the DSM-5.

Since 2012 there has been a concerted effort by an international consortium of academics and clinicians to develop a systematic review of all aspects of DCD, from the definition, assessment, diagnosis and intervention to underlying processes (Blank et al. 2019). We address its recommendations, particularly in the intervention section of the book, as detailed analyses of all meta-studies have been undertaken in this area. Ongoing work has been published on recommendations so far (Blank et al. 2012, 2019) with further developments yet to be published and at the Eleventh World DCD conference held in Toulouse in 2015. The most recent work on this was at the International Consensus meeting in Stockholm in May/June 2016, culminating in the Blank et al. (2019) guidelines. It is expected that recommendations from this recent document will be adopted worldwide.

The clinical implications and processes of assessment and diagnosis aligned to these recommendations are detailed in Chapters 4 and 6.

*Co-occurring characteristics in DCD*

The core defining characteristic of DCD is motor in nature, but as in any developmental disorders it is not the only characteristic. In probably over 50% of cases there will be some co-occurring characteristics, namely deficits in attention, literacy, cognition, social, emotional functioning and language. These are labelled in their own right as ADHD, dyslexia, ASD and DLD. Thus, there are two interlocking bodies of literature that describe these children. The first describes children with DCD as showing movement difficulties as their primary diagnosis and how most of them exhibit co-occurring characteristics. The second describes the developmental disorders noted above and notes that the prevalence of movement difficulties in these children is higher than that in their typically developing, matched peers. The literature sources that chronicle co-occurring characteristics include the following: Kaplan et al. 1998, 2006; Kadesjo and Gillberg 1999; Skinner and Piek 2001; Gillberg and Kadesjo 2003; Green and Baird 2005; Lingham et al. 2009; Blank et al. 2019. The co-occurring difficulties are important for two reasons. First, it is probable that the majority of the children with DCD have a co-occurring condition and ignoring it would give an incomplete view of their condition. Second, co-occurring difficulties need to be considered when developing intervention strategies. For example, when support and intervention strategies are being developed, a child with DCD and attention problems will require a different approach to one who has only a movement difficulty.

*Progression of DCD*

Some of the historical literature on DCD stated that children grow out of the condition because it was seen as a temporary difficulty that with maturation and growth would go away. However, other studies have shown that this is not the case and that without intervention, the difficulties often continue from early childhood, through to adolescence, into emerging adulthood (Losse et al.1991; Cantell et al. 1994, 2003; Rasmussen and Gillberg 2000; Piek 2003; Missiuna et al. 2007; Blank et al. 2019. What we do know is that parents and the individuals concerned change in their perception and views as to what is most important. In the early years, the motor skills are the foremost concern of parents, focusing on motor related activities of daily living and play activities (Missiuna et al. 2007). Concerns continue about types of recreational activities during later childhood and changes again in emerging adulthood. In a series of articles, Kirby et al. have shown that not only do the motor characteristics, in the main, continue but that other attributes are affected (Kirby et al. 2008a, b, 2010, 2011). In terms of the central motor component, Kirby et al. (2011) have shown that adults diagnosed in childhood with DCD have coordination difficulties and that these affect activities in later life, such as driving. These individuals do not have a higher prevalence of serious accidents, but they have more 'minor ones', such as hitting gateposts; it is as though they are aware of their limitations. Kirby et al. (2011) also speculate that motor difficulties diagnosed in a child with DCD include impairment in such as planning and organization, which, in turn, may severely influence and restrict their social interactions.

*Prevalence of DCD*

The DSM-5 provides an estimated prevalence of DCD of around 5% to 6% in children aged 7 years, specifying 1.8% as severe and 3% as probable. The male-female ratio is estimated to be between 2:1 and 7:1 (Blank et al. 2019). However, as with all prevalence figures, this ratio depends on the criteria used to determine it. While prevalence figures between 5% and 20% have been estimated, prevalences of 5% to 6% are most frequently reported (Gaines et al. 2008). Higher figures, in our opinion, tend to be pragmatic estimates rather than based on actual data from studies. Prevalence becomes important, however, if, as in some countries, support can only be obtained after an official diagnosis. In other countries, a child can receive assistance in a graded manner without a formal diagnosis, through education and health services. This is addressed in Chapter 7.

A detailed examination of DCD prevalence was provided by Lingham et al. (2009) from data on 7000 children aged 7 years of age as part of the Avon Longitudinal Study of Parents and Children. Addressing all four criteria from DSM-IV (APA 2000) they presented a conservative prevalence figure of 1.7% and a second of 4.9%. They concluded that the former figure would represent identifiable DCD and the latter as probable DCD. This was an important study because of the large numbers involved. They used subtests of the Movement Assessment Battery for Children (MABC) to examine for Criterion A in the DSM-IV definition, a handwriting and parent questionnaire for Criterion B, available neurological information for Criterion C and the Wechsler Intelligence Scale for Children for Criterion D. Their figures are similar to those found by Wright and Sugden (1996) using a two-step approach to diagnosis, involving a standardized test (MABC Test) and the MABC Checklist, which together address criteria A and B, with C and D (DSM-IV) also being included in this study.

Other studies have found a higher prevalence, and when examining prevalence, it is prudent to look at the criteria used. As a coarse-grained recommendation, we would agree with an estimate of around 5% to 6% for a definitive diagnosis, but any diagnoses should be based on the collation of information from a variety of sources. The guidelines from the MABC-2 use 5% prevalence for those needing immediate attention and 15% for monitoring those at risk. Again, this is based on custom and practice and, of course, only examines Criteria A and B of the DSM-IV criteria using the MABC Test and Checklist and so is only part of any diagnostic process.

With respect to sex differences in DCD, there are a variety of figures, but the majority show a higher male prevalence, with ratios ranging from 1.7:1 (Lingham et al. 2009) to much higher figures up to 7.0:1 (Blank et al. 2019). Much of the discrepancy in sex ratios is probably due to the tests employed to diagnose the disorder. In this regard, it is prudent to examine the cut off points in the criteria of the methods and the methods employed. The reasons for this sex imbalance are unclear, This imbalance is also found in other developmental disorders, such ASD and ADHD, to varying degrees. It is often explained by females presenting in a different, less obvious manner than males. This may account for the apparent underestimation.

*Causes and epidemiology of DCD*

A possible model of causality has been presented by Morton (2004) with reference to overall developmental disorders. If one looks at this with reference to DCD, the causes of DCD can reside in either a biological or cognitive framework that affects the behavioural characteristics. There are some speculative biological causes, such as those alluding to some form of brain damage or malfunction. From earlier studies on minimal brain damage to more recent ones on atypical brain development (Kaplan et al. 1998) and minor neurological deficit (Hadders-Algra 2003), there has been a constant search for underlying biological substrates. If any of these atypical brain functions are found to be the cause of DCD, it will raise an important paradox or conundrum, because Criterion D of the DSM criteria says that the condition should then be excluded. At the moment, the science is not available to firmly establish atypical brain functions, although magnetic resonance imaging techniques are giving us better insights in to the workings of the brain; however, direct relationships between brain and behaviour are not yet totally clear. (Kagerer et al. 2006; Cantin et al. 2007). Ongoing work that is proving to be exciting is that of Zwicker et al. (2009, 2010) and (Wilson et al. 2018), who are looking at cognitive and neural correlates in DCD.

As one moves from the biological to more cognitive and perceptual processes, other pathways emerge. Both vision and kinaesthesis have been proposed as possible causative factors, with both areas providing information for fruitful discussion. The early work of Jean Ayres (1979) on sensorimotor functions has spawned a whole area of explanation and intervention schedules, much of which will be discussed in Chapters 5, 6 and 7. For now, it is pertinent to note that several studies, noted by Mon-Williams et al. (1999), have provided evidence showing that children with DCD are poorer at visual–kinaesthetic cross-modal matching than their peers. This does not necessarily provide a causal relationship. Reaction times have traditionally been recorded as slower in children with DCD, possibly with some of the complex paradigms showing a lack of flexibility of responses in children with DCD. Wilson et al., with novel experiments on internal modelling, have shown that children with DCD have an impaired ability to internally represent action, providing a further route and explanation of the cognitive and neural aspects of DCD (Wilson et al. 2004, 2013, 2014, 2018). Further development of the work from this group appears to be promising in the quest to understand the underlying causes.

Caution is advised here, as a higher prevalence of a particular ability, such as kinaesthesis or visual perception, does not imply causation. Indeed, when we measure many of the underlying processes of movement production in children with DCD, although we do find a higher prevalence than in typical developing children, it is the totality of

> **Box 1.3** Summary on DCD
>
> ✓ The core difficulty in DCD is impairment in the learning and performance of motor skills affecting activities of daily living and/or academic achievement.
> ✓ It is developmental and, with or without support, many difficulties continue into adulthood.
> ✓ Prevalence is around 5% to 6% for those requiring immediate attention and up to 15% for those to be monitored for DCD.
> ✓ It is usually accompanied by associated characteristics.
> ✓ Possible causes are numerous, ranging from constitutional problems to environmental circumstances.
> ✓ The condition is not better explained by other named disabilities, such as cerebral palsy or muscular dystrophy.

the difficulties experienced rather than one specific attribute that points to the motor problems (see Box 1.3).

A recent paper by Wade and Kazek (2017) has challenged the conventional approaches to causation of internal models of information processing and executive function ideas as explanations of the basic poor coordination feature of DCD. Executive function is a multifaceted concept involving planning, organization, freedom from distraction, short-term memory and other cognitive processes, and is often noted as a co-occurring feature of DCD. Wade and Kazek (2017) propose a different explanation, favouring a dynamical systems explanation concentrating on perception action links and how the organism and the affordances in the environment transact to produce the end result. This is elaborated in later chapters. The journal (Human Movement Science) invited comments on the Wade and Kazek article; one noted that there are several publications that attest to a more neurological basis to DCD (Wilson et al. 2018). The debate on how DCD can be explained, whether by internal neurological models or by more ecological ones, emphasizing the role of context, will continue and the evidence emerging over the next few years should give us a much clearer picture. Blank et al. (2019) note that there appears to be evidence that motor control difficulties in DCD depend on which tasks the individual is performing and the demands made by these in situations that involve dual tasks, for example. We would agree with this, adding again that the unit of analysis is always the individual in context, not solely the individual.

More research on DCD is needed in two specific areas. The first is in learning of motor tasks. If we accept that a child's current motoric competence is a result of learning, either through experience or more directed teaching and therapy, then more learning studies are required. There is a dearth of such studies at the moment, and although one may argue that intervention studies are in the area of learning, more strictly controlled studies are needed that can unearth in detail the underlying processes. A second area that would enhance our knowledge of DCD is the area of 'coordination'. The label of the condition is developmental *coordination* disorder and yet coordination per se is not as frequently studied as we would like. At the World DCD Conference in Lausanne in 2013, Karl Newell, a renowned scholar in motor learning, alluded to the absence of studies on coordination considering that it was in the title of the condition! Wade and Kazek (2017) and the Wilson group in Australia go some way to redressing this balance (see Wilson et al. 2018) but there are few other studies about DCD that look directly at coordination dynamics.

## Other developmental disorders

Below we present the definitions and diagnostic recommendations of other selected developmental disorders from the DSM-5 (see Box 1.4). Motor difficulties are an important part of the profile of many children, but the motor difficulties are not a core feature or the diagnosis. There is strong evidence showing that in these children there is a higher prevalence of such difficulties than one would find in their typically developing peers. What follows is a synopsis and description of each of these conditions with more detail about their motor difficulties outside of the core diagnosis. Children with these developmental disorders will show more co-occurring characteristics than their peers, with motor performance being one of them.

Explanations for developmental disorders are many, but we have found the model from Morton (2004) to be most helpful for our understanding. In this model, Morton encourages us to consider the difficulties and explanations for the difficulties seen in developmental disorders in different ways. Specifically, he splits behaviour (what we see/measure) from cognition and biology, with cognition seen as an intervening variable between the biological

---

**Box 1.4** Common developmental disorders

✓ **Dyslexia** is associated with the literacy skills of reading, writing and spelling. Shortcomings in phonological processes, working memory and processing speed are common features. (Note: in the DSM-5 it is listed under Specific Learning Disorders with a specific note on impairment in reading. Throughout this text we use the more common term dyslexia).

✓ **Autism spectrum disorder** describes some children who are severely impaired across a wide range of functioning – language, social, motor, cognitive and other areas – for whom low cognitive ability is not a characteristic, but their social and personal skills still make communication, interaction and daily functioning very difficult.

✓ **Attention–deficit–hyperactivity disorder** has as its core characteristic an impaired attentional system that may or may not be accompanied by hyperactivity.

✓ **Developmental language disorder** involves a difficulty with expressive and/or receptive language often appearing to be out of line with overall functioning in other domains.

**Biology**

**Dyslexia    Autism    ADHD    DLD    DCD**

Brain functions; neurology; genetic determination

**Cognitive Processes**

General information processing variables e.g. attention, memory, executive function, planning

Phonological deficit    Theory of mind    Executive functioning    Language coordination

Empathy-systemizing

**Behaviour**

| Reading, spelling & writing difficulties | Poor social skills Rigidity of response | Attention, impulsivity, hyperactivity difficulties | Receptive/expressive language difficulties | Clumsiness |

**Figure 1.2** Adaptation of the Morton (2004) model showing examples from five developmental disorders. ADHD, attention-deficit–hyperactivity disorder: DLD, developmental language disorder; DCD, developmental coordination disorder.

make-up of the child and the resultant behaviour. He presents a model for autism using these constructs and we have adapted this model to hypothesize how biology, cognition and behaviour link to developmental disorders, including DCD (Fig. 1.2). The model shows that the intervening variables involving cognition may be common across the five disorders, making it likely that they have similarities in co-occurring conditions, such as the motor problems present in DCD.

*Dyslexia*

Dyslexia is a disorder that seems to generate huge interest among professionals and others. Both the American Psychiatric Association and the World Health Organization (1992) *International Statistical Classification of Diseases and Related Health Problems*, 10th edition refer to characteristics that may be classed as dyslexia, although they are called by other titles such as specific learning disorder (DSM-5). At its fundamental level the term generally refers to a difficulty in reading, writing or spelling. The DSM-5 notes characteristics that include 'inaccurate or slow and effortful reading … difficulty in understanding the meaning of what is read … difficulties in spelling … difficulties with written expression' (DSM-5 2013, p. 66). There is great debate about several issues within this field. One is the 'discrepancy' notion, which states that literacy skills are out of line with other attributes, such as intelligence (DSM-5). Another is the difference, if any, between children with dyslexia and others who have reading or literacy difficulties but are not described as dyslexic. These and other controversies are well discussed in books by Hulme and Snowling (2009) and by Elliott and Grigorenko (2014).

There is some consensus about many of the characteristics, for example, the noted difficulty in literacy, particularly reading. If one invokes a discrepancy notion, then this difficulty is unexpected. However, in line with our other comments on developmental disorders, we would always recommend focusing on the profile of the children and their strengths and needs. Often in the early years, language is a problem that can lead to a central difficulty in phonological processing, which has been proposed as a fundamental aspect of dyslexia (Hulme and Snowling 2009). Other reported difficulties include speed of processing, working memory and various perceptual tasks. In the early years, the phonological mapping of speech sounds to words seemed to predominate, with this later becoming more focused on meaning and fluency.

The search for biological substrates has been a constant endeavour with genetic studies (Cope et al. 2005; Harold et al. 2006), twin studies (De Fries and Alarcon 1996) and indeed social and classroom experiences (Rutter and Maughan 2002) being undertaken. Because of the similarities and possible overlap between children with dyslexia and others with an unnamed reading disorder, the question arises as to whether dyslexia is a categorical diagnosis. Is there a distinct line between children with dyslexia and children with other reading disorders, or is this a continuum of reading problems, with different parts of the continuum manifesting slightly different characteristics?

There has been a long history of looking at motor problems in this group of individuals. Classic work from Orton (1937) and Rutter and Yule (1975), together with work in Canada during the 1990s looked at large groups of children to get a better understanding of developmental disorders as a whole (Kaplan et al. 1997). The Kaplan et al. study involved 224 children with reading difficulties between the ages of 8 and 16 years and matched to 155 peers. Of the children with reading difficulties, 27% were also diagnosed as having motor difficulties. This type of overlap was not unexpected.

The overlap of motor and reading difficulties has led to the proposal by Nicolson et al. (2001) of an automatization deficit hypothesis coming from their work on dual tasks. From this work, they proposed that the problem lay in the cerebellum that led to the literacy difficulties and linking it to other tasks involving motor processes, such as balance, thereby establishing a link between motor and reading processes. This has been well debated in the literature with differing conclusions (Yap and van der Leij 1994; Bishop 2007) (see Box 1.5).

**Box 1.5** Summary on dyslexia

✓ Core difficulties are in the areas of reading, writing and spelling.
✓ There is debate as to the differences between dyslexia and regular reading difficulties.
✓ There is debate as to whether to include a discrepancy between reading ability and overall ability in the diagnostic process.
✓ Underlying causation includes phonological difficulties, working memory and speed of processing.

The link between motor ability and dyslexia has been shown in numerous ways and, clearly again, there is a higher prevalence of children in this group with motor difficulties than there is in a typically developing group.

### Autism spectrum disorder

This most interesting and fascinating of conditions has been observed since the middle ages but came to the fore through the work of both Kanner (1943) in the USA and Asperger (1944) in Germany. As the term 'autistic spectrum disorder' suggests, there is a spectrum of characteristics and features that have at the core a problem with cognition and socialization.

The DSM-5 provides the diagnostic criteria of ASD, and it is pertinent to note here the latest edition combines classic autism and Asperger syndrome into one spectrum or continuum.

The DSM-5 criteria include persistent problems in social communication in different social contexts. This is shown in Criterion A that notes impaired reciprocity during normal dialogue and impaired sharing of emotions. The criteria would also include atypical body language, facial expression and reduced eye contact. This in turn contributes to problems in relationships and spontaneous adjustments to the demands of different social situations. Criterion B involves stereotypical and repetitive movements with speech or objects, a rigidity where sameness is insisted upon and a highly restricted set of interests, often with an abnormal intensity of attachment. In many cases, there are reports of an unusual response to sensory input that can be manifested in either hypo- or hypersensitivity. These symptoms are present early in the developmental period and cause significant impairment in various areas of everyday functioning. As with other developmental disorders, the symptoms are not better explained by intellectual difficulties or global developmental delay.

There have been a number of theories that have been offered as explanations of the condition from a cognitive viewpoint. These include theory of mind (Baron-Cohen et al. 1985), central coherence theory (Frith 1989), executive function (Hill 2004) and empathy–systemizing (Baron-Cohen 2008, 2010). More recently, others (Mottron et al. 2014) argue for what they call a 'trigger threshold target brain plasticity' model to explain autism characteristics. All of these are proposed as intervening and mediating variables between brain differences and the observed behaviour. Individuals on the autism spectrum have a wide range of abilities ranging from those who have severe difficulties with language and communication, to those called 'high functioning', who show special abilities in fields such as art, music and mathematics, for example. Yet this group would still exhibit the core characteristics of the condition.

When we examine the motor performance of children with ASD, again we find a much higher prevalence of those with motor difficulties compared to typically developing peers. Green et al. (2009) have noted that children with DCD have been shown to have characteristics of ASD and vice versa. In a group of children with Asperger syndrome Miyahara (1994) found over 80% scored below the 5th centile on the MABC Test. A similar result was found by Green et al. (2002). In addition, Jansiewicz et al. (2006) found that children with ASD also exhibit atypical movements, such as walking on the outside of their feet or associated movements often viewed as neurological soft sign indicators. Others have reported 'clumsy gait', slow reactions and response speeds, early crawling and walking difficulties and motor praxis problems, as indicated by imitation of gesture tests (Hallet et al. 1993; Teitelbaum et al. 1998; Noterdaeme et al. 2002; Jansiewicz et al. 2006). The motor praxis problem has been suggested to be a consequence of problems in joint attention or a poor mirror neuron system (Rogers et al. 1996; Mostofsky et al. 2007, 2009). Green et al. (2009) in their study of 101 children with ASD found 80 below the 5th centile of the MABC, 10 between the 5th and 15th centile and 11 with no problem. Crucial to this study is that, of those in a low IQ group, 97% had movement difficulties and exhibited lower scores on the MABC than the higher IQ group. Therefore, intellectual difficulty may be a major contributing factor. Thus, here we have a confounding variable of intelligence, in that individuals with a low IQ may not understand the instructions to complete a test item for the MABC, as we know that in any group of children with an IQ below 70, the prevalence of motor difficulties increases greatly. The Green et al. (2009) study noted that although IQ was a factor it did not account for the total poor performance of the children and went on to show that complexity of the task, in this case timing demands, may be a factor. Overall, it is clear that across the autistic spectrum, individuals show a greatly increased prevalence of motor disorders. We are unsure of the reasons for this, but suggest that biological, cognitive and environmental factors may contribute. If we

---

**Box 1.6** Summary on autism spectrum disorder

✓ As the name suggests, ASD is a spectrum ranging from mild to severe involvement and low to high IQs. The former Asperger label is no longer included in DSM-5, with these individuals now labelled as having ASD, i.e. being on the general autism spectrum.

✓ Persistent problems in social communication across different social contexts.

✓ Individuals exhibit stereotypical and repetitive actions.

✓ Problems present early in life and cause difficulties in normal day-to-day interactive functioning.

✓ Explanations include atypical theory of mind, central coherence theory, executive functioning, empathy-systemizing and trigger threshold target.

✓ Affected children occasionally have special abilities.

✓ Clumsiness and other motor difficulties are often seen in this group with the degree often being specifically related to the extent and severity of autism.

could change the environment in ways that would facilitate participation and implement good teaching and therapy in a dynamic manner with our interventions, we would be better able to support these children.

A recent systematic review confirms that children with ASD and DCD share some characteristics (Cacola et al. 2017). However, it is also reported that they do not have similar profiles and the conditions can be separated with distinct distributions.

### Attention-deficit–hyperactivity disorder

The essential features of ADHD/ADD are that the individual shows persistent patterns of inattention and/or hyperactivity that interfere with daily function or development. The DSM-5 lists nine symptoms of **inattention** of which six or more must be present, are at odds with the developmental level of the individual and interfere with daily functioning. Examples of these include failing to give close attention to detail or making careless mistakes, difficulty organizing tasks and activities, having messy work and difficulty sustaining attention. The DSM-5 also lists nine symptoms of **hyperactivity and impulsivity,** which again are inconsistent with developmental level and are not due to other conditions such as oppositional behaviour disorder. Such behaviours would include fidgeting or squirming with hands or feet, running around in inappropriate situations, answering a question before full information is given and difficulty waiting turn. For a full list of these symptoms for both inattention and hyperactivity/impulsivity see DSM-5 (pp. 59–60). The condition should have been apparent before the age of 12 years, and the characteristics are present in two or more settings – school, home, or workplace. The symptoms also have an adverse effect on schoolwork or occupation, and are not better explained by another condition such as schizophrenia. Three types of ADHD are specified: hyperactive/impulsive, inattentive and a combination of hyperactive/impulsive and inattentive.

It is not surprising that individuals with ADHD are reported to have a number of co-occurring difficulties. Attention is a major attribute and a deficit in this area can lead to a host of difficulties, including those involving motor actions. Similarly, a person who is impulsive or hyperactive may show a lack of motoric control by either moving too quickly, and/or at the wrong time. In the framework of Morton (2004) that illustrates biological substrates, and cognitive deficits affecting behaviour, the most common explanation of cognitive underpinning is that of executive control. This involves response inhibition, working memory and planning and organization, set and task shifting and interference control (Barkley 1997; Hulme and Snowling 2009). It is no coincidence that these abilities are the ones that are listed by some professionals as being problematic in children with DCD. This is not only found in the seemingly more obvious gross motor skills, but also in handwriting (Pereira et al. 2000). Relationships between DCD and ADHD have been noted by authors such as

> **Box 1.7** Summary on attention-deficit–hyperactivity disorder
>
> ✓ Involves persistent patterns of inattention and/or hyperactivity across multiple contexts.
> ✓ Should be seen clearly before the age of 12.
> ✓ Includes impulsivity, restlessness, running around inappropriately, difficulty waiting turn, persistent daydreaming.
> ✓ Can lead to several other difficulties such as underachievement and behavioural difficulties.
> ✓ Causes include poor executive function, involving inadequate response inhibition, planning and working memory difficulties.
> ✓ The above characteristics are related to a group that, overall, has mild motor difficulties (DSM-5).

Kadesjo and Gillberg 1999; Ramussen and Gillberg 2000; Tseng et al. 2004; Kaplan et al. 2006. For a more comprehensive review of the link between ADHD and motor problems see Sugden and Wade (2013). The generic summary is that problems in impulse control, inattention and hyperactivity either are, or can be, related to motor difficulties. Whether these are causing the motor difficulties or whether the causation is the other way around is unclear, but there is a strong link.

*Developmental language disorder*
Most of the definitions of speech and language problems involve a discrepancy in that it is often stated that these problems are out of line with other areas of ability, such as intelligence. In the DSM-5, a diagnosis involves both a standardized IQ test and a language test, with the impairment being diagnosed when there is a significant discrepancy between the two and with the speech and language scores being lower than IQ scores, often by two standard deviations. The International Classification of Diseases (ICD 1; WHO 1992) criteria are often used in diagnosis of DLD, with three areas considered: speech articulation disorder, expressive language disorder and receptive language disorder. In children with DLD it is noted that a usual precursor to the condition is a delay in onset and slow development of early language.

Speech articulation problems involve a significant delay or impairment in the ability to pronounce speech sounds correctly. It can occur with or without expressive or receptive language difficulties. Often there are idiosyncratic patterns in addition to the slowness and delay. Expressive language disorder involves difficulties in the use of language compared with peers and overlaps with articulation disorders about 40% of the time. Prevalence rates of both these are around 3%, depending on measurement with the male–female sex ratio of between 2 and 5 to 1. Receptive language involves impairment in understanding language, again being out of line with the child's intelligence as measured by other means. Prevalence is again around 2%, with a male–female ratio of between 2–4 to 1 (Johnson and Beitchman 2006).

The causes of DLD range from specific impaired linguistic systems (favoured by linguists), with the core issue being a problem with the knowledge of grammar. This view regards language as being separate from other cognitive functions. On the other hand, some psychologists tend to favour more generic cognitive explanations, with processes operating in a more cooperative way with other areas of cognition, and not specific to problems of grammar (Hulme and Snowling 2009).

The link between speech, in particular, and language in general with movement is one that is not difficult to make. Iverson (2010) for example examines language development in a child, and the role of motor development in particular, in providing the opportunity to practice skills relevant to language before they are required for that purpose. This is very similar to the more general development study by Campos et al. (2000) entitled *Travel Broadens the Mind* mentioned earlier, which notes that motor development facilitates the development of other attributes.

At a global level one can say that the action of speech involves movement, such as in verbal dyspraxia, and movement itself in the form of gestures and body language does involve some form of communication. If one delves deeper into the areas of language and movement, one finds that there is also commonality in that they are both generative. In other words, it is possible to transmit meaning in several different ways when speaking by using different words and phrases, yet still make the same point. In a similar manner, when moving one can perform different actions to achieve the same results, such as picking up an object. Thus, one can conclude that it is not surprising that children with speech and language difficulties often show other movement problems. A review of the link between language impairment and motor abilities was undertaken by Hill (2001). She noted that there may be underlying common brain areas and genetic factors may also play a role (Bishop 2002). Several studies have pointed to children with DLD performing poorly on motor tests or actions. Powell and Bishop (1992) found this and proposed that it could be due to one or more of three factors: left hemisphere difficulties, slow rate of processing, or imperfect visual processing. They concluded that only imperfect visual processing seemed to be a promising explanation. In a series of tasks involving gestures, Hill (1998) showed that children with DCD and those with DLD were poorer on some of the tests, but it was only in meaningful gestures and not on copying unfamiliar hand postures. Both groups were poorer than their age-matched peers and similar to younger, typically developing children.

Movement and language are similar in many ways, with a major aspiration being the solving of novel problems whether language or motor based. In addition, in a sample of children with DLD we will find a higher prevalence of children with movement difficulties. But as is the case with the other developmental disorders, this is simply an increase in prevalence, not a one to one correspondence, nor one that should be used for prediction.

**Box 1.8** Summary on developmental language disorder

✓ Problems in either or both receptive and expressive language.

✓ Usually there is a discrepancy difference between communication skills and the overall ability of the child.

✓ Prevalence is around 3%, depending upon criteria, with males at least twice as prevalent as females.

✓ Causes involve both specific impaired linguistic systems to more general cognitive and biological explanations.

✓ Poor motor functioning has been linked to both biological brain factors and those involving cognition.

## Case studies

We present two case studies: the first is for DCD and the second for other developmental disorders. Both have been developed from numerous profiles we have observed in clinical settings and demonstrate the traditional presentations of the disorders. In later chapters (see Chapter 7) we describe and follow through in detail six different case studies of DCD and other developmental disorders.

**Case Study: DCD**

*Jason is 9 years old and his teachers and parents have noted that he has several needs that require attention. He is one of a family of four with two older sisters and a younger brother. He had a typical birth and in his first year of life he seemed to be developing as his sisters had done. He was a little late in some of his motoric milestones, but not so different as to cause concern. However, by the time he was 2 years old, it was clear that progression had not been made as expected. His gait was awkward; he was not close to running and he had difficulty with manipulating objects. At 5 years of age the gap between his and typical expectancies had widened; and as the environmental demands increased so his performance was noticeably lower than his peers.*

*In the first year of school his writing and drawing skills were poor. He had difficulty with letter formation and his copying of shapes was also not up to expectation. His grip was awkward, which made it difficult for him to write quickly when necessary. It was also noticeable that he did not appear to have the necessary fundamental gross motor skills that allowed him to participate appropriately in recreational activities.*

*As he progressed through primary school Jason received different types of instructions to improve his writing skills and this seemed to confuse him and set him back further in this area. His reading was at age appropriate level and his other academic skills gave no real cause for concern, other than that he could not write much of what he knew. His verbal responses in class were satisfactory.*

*In the playground and in physical education (PE) lessons Jason had great difficulties. He still showed problems in running and looked awkward with arms and legs seemingly not being coordinated with each other and moving almost independently. This often led to him being teased by his classmates. His ball skills were also poor, and he seemed frightened when a ball was thrown to him; it is not clear whether this was because he knew he would have difficulty catching it. His lack of skills in this area kept him separate from his peers. He was excluded from games in the playground and he had no real recreational interests outside of school. He spent much of his time in his room listening to music; he was very knowledgeable about jazz. His parents have encouraged this interest and he has started taking saxophone lessons and practices with gusto. He has just finished his first-grade examination on this instrument.*

*Jason cannot ride a bicycle and he has given up trying to learn. This in turn leaves him isolated from friends when they are playing out after school or during the holidays. He is still slow to dress and slow in other self-care activities, which further restricts his social interaction and makes things difficult for him when he is getting dressed and undressed for PE. He was assessed on the MABC Test and Checklist (Henderson et al. 2007) and scored below the 10th centile on both.*

*His parents and teachers feel that Jason's motor skills are not only hindering the progress of this averagely intelligent boy, but also are also severely restricting his social interaction with his peers. He is not unruly in class, although his attention wanders a little and he has few friends. His parents and teachers all feel that support is required to try to remedy his poor movement skills and have initiated the process of linking his assessments to intervention protocols. Jason is a likeable boy who tries hard and can at times persevere at practicing various motor activities.*

**Comment:** Jason is typical of some of the children we see who have movement difficulties. These difficulties not only interfere with his participation in movement activities that surround him in daily life, but they also have a negative influence on other areas such as friendships. Any programme of intervention and support should naturally include activities that involve both 'learning to move' and 'moving to learn'. The former involves learning and developing the capacity to perform successfully numerous specific skills that occur in everyday life and being able to approach novel movement situations with confidence. The second involves using movement as a facilitator for other skills such as cooperation and confidence.

Jason is also an example of the children who show movement difficulties as a primary characteristic that appear to be affecting other areas of their functioning, such as social interaction. A support programme with some learning to move and moving to learn activities would be recommended. Different and more detailed case studies are presented in Chapter 3 and these are taken through some of the following chapters illustrating possibilities for support and intervention.

## Case Study: Other neurodevelopmental disorders

The case study of Alice presented below shows the type of pupil we often see. Alice shows a range of difficulties, but she has not had a formal diagnosis of any named condition. However, her attention seems to be impaired, which can lead to other difficulties in the school. Poor social interaction is another of her problems again possibly leading to underachievement.

*Alice is a 12-year-old girl in mainstream school who is shy and has difficulty in interacting with her classmates. Her attention tends to wander in class. Her schoolwork is average but her attentional difficulties and lack of social interaction give her teachers and parents cause for concern. There has been no official diagnosis of any named condition, but attention-deficit disorder has been mentioned by both parents and teachers. She is a 'dreamer' in class but shows no problem in terms of hyperactivity or other behaviour problems. The teachers constantly refer to her as underachieving because of her lack of attention, and this problem has increased since her move from primary to secondary school. In secondary school she forgets her homework and often fails to note what she is supposed to do. She gets 'lost' in the school and often asks classmates what the teacher has just instructed. In terms of attention, she appears to have difficulty in coming to attention, in selecting the important things to concentrate on. She has a short attention span when on task and is easily distracted.*

*Alice also has significant movement difficulties. When walking and running she looks 'awkward'. Her parents note that she has rarely involved herself in recreational activities. She was late walking and hardly ever played the usual children's games with her friends. She has difficulty riding a bicycle and her parents consider that she is not competent enough to ride on public roads. Her handwriting is slow but neat as is her texting, which is slow but with few errors.*

*Alice is a very quiet girl who is no trouble in school. She is an average reader and her work is neat but slow. She wants to please, but her social interaction skills are not good enough for her to make real friends. Movement is not the main difficulty for Alice; her main problems appear to be with attention and social interaction. But these are co-occurring characteristics are part of the overall profile of her abilities and aptitudes that hinder her ability and lead to a lack of participation in leisure and recreational activities. These along with her immature social skills, leave her with few friends.*

**Comment:** Alice presents a number of challenges that we often see in children who have a range of difficulties, but who have not had a formal diagnosis of any named condition. However, her attention seems to be impaired and which can lead to other difficulties in the school. Poor social interaction is another of her problems again possibly leading to underachievement.

Any programme of support should address her attention difficulties but in the context of meaningful and enjoyable activities. Alice's choices, both in and out of the classroom. These would include movement activities and the use of these to learn attentional skills. A programme for this type of profile is shown in Chapter 7.

## Assessing types of movement difficulties

It is usual when examining movement difficulties to simply look at the characteristics of the children or groups of children. This can be done in an observational manner by parents and family members who note that gross motor skills are poor and that fine motor skills are within a range of typical variation. We as professionals do this every day, noting the motor achievements of children, whether the early milestones or later when children are acquiring their fundamental movement skills. The DSM-5 classifies early milestones as knife and fork usage, dressing skills and later ones such as puzzle assembly, handwriting and playing ball games. This type of analysis through observation is enhanced by reports from professionals such as occupational therapists, physiother-apists and teachers. These observations are as important as the more standardized tests and should be used in conjunction with them.

Another way to examine patterns is to see how children score on a particular recog-nized assessment instrument such as the MABC and use its structure. The MABC has three sections in the Test and three in the Checklist. The Test contains the sections on Manual Dexterity, Aiming and Catching and Balance with each section comprising two or three items. The Checklist contains three sections: movement in a static and/or pre-dictable environment; movement in a dynamic and/or unpredictable environment; and non-motor factors that might affect movement. Thus, one can obtain an overall score of impairment together with specific scores in the sections of the Test or Checklist. Such tests are only one way of building a profile of movement difficulties, but each result is dependent upon the validity of the instrument in question.

Examining how profiles of movement abilities have been described in typically developing children using statistical techniques such as factor analysis, is a method that can be used to determine whether all children with movement difficulties follow the same patterns.

### Movement profiles in typically developing children
Movement abilities have been classified in typical populations across the movement domain using the statistical procedures of factor and cluster analysis. These are mathematical procedures that calculate commonality across various tests and individuals employing correlations Those that are highly correlated with each other form a 'factor' or 'cluster'. Thus, to classify movement abilities in a typical population, a sample of individuals is assessed on various tests and the results correlated with each other and analysed to see how the tasks cluster together forming 'factors'. Each factor will have a strength according to how high the correlations are, and each factor is given a name by the experimenter. Large groups are assessed on numerous tests and those with high correlations with each other form a factor. In this way, the number of factors is very much less than the original number of tests. Probably the most comprehensive study in children using this method was conducted in the 1970s by Larry Rarick and colleagues at the University of California at Berkeley. He followed the methodology used by Fleishman in 1964. Rarick et al. (1976) tested 145 typically developing children aged 6 years and aged 9–13 years old. Boys and girls were analysed separately, but six common factors were identified in both sexes: gross limb coordination; strength, power and body size; fine-visual-motor coordination; fat or dead weight; balance and leg power and coordination. These six factors accounted for around 70% of the total variance in both boys and girls. Rarick et al. (1976) also examined factor structures in children with intellectual disabilities.

More recently, Schultz et al. (2011) performed confirmatory factor analysis on the data from the MABC (Henderson et al. 2007). This study was for the purpose of examining the structure of the MABC. Data from 1172 children across three age bands were used. The findings were that in the younger age group (3–6y) a complex factor emerged with a general overall factor as well as specific factors for the three components of the test. This general factor disappeared with age, with only modest correlations between each factor. The authors interpreted this data as confirmation of the differentiation of abilities as the child develops. A cautionary note is that this study was not examining factor structure of movement in children's motor abilities per se but was a confirmatory factor study of the components of the assessment instrument the MABC-2. Nevertheless, it does help us identify certain traits in children's development, with this one pointing to a move from more general abilities to ones that are differentiated. In another study looking at the reliability and validity of factors in the MABC-2 age band 2 in a Japanese sample, there was acceptable internal consistence and high factorial validity (Kita et al. 2016).

*Movement in children with developmental coordination disorder*
Several studies (mainly using factor and cluster analysis techniques) have examined subgroups in children with DCD. One of the earlier studies found children with the following five clusters (Hoare 1994):

1. Low performance on kinaesthetic acuity and running.

2. Low scores on kinaesthetic acuity and balance.

3. Overall low scores but biased towards perceptual tasks.

4. More specific low visual scores.

5. Good perceptual scores but low motor execution.

These factors point to some fundamental perceptual problems that probably reinforced the early emphasis on remediation in that area. Macnab et al. (2001) came close to replicating this in children showing more severe difficulties.

Other studies have concentrated more on the motor aspect of the condition. Sugden and Wright (1996, 1998) used the eight subcomponents of the MABC Test (Henderson and Sugden 1992) together with the four sections of the MABC Checklist. Factor analysis was followed by cluster analysis and produced the following four final clusters:

1. Children with moderate difficulties across the range of skills.

2. Children specifically with catching difficulties.

3. Children who had difficulties in adjusting their movements to the movement of others or the environment.

4. Children with specific manual skills difficulties.

More recently, Rivard et al. (2014) using the Developmental Coordination Disorder Questionnaire (DCDQ) in a population-based sample, found a three-factor solution. The study was completed on 3151 children between the ages of 8 and 15 years. The study found that 73 boys and 49 girls met the DCD criteria. The larger sample group was used for factor analysis with the three factors – control during movement, fine motor and handwriting and general coordination – in total accounting for around 70% of the variance. Individually they accounted for 33%, 25% and 13%, respectively.

This study confirmed Visser's (2007) view that a generalized problem is often found and that other difficulties are probably dependent on the tests that are fed into the factor and cluster analyses. As we become more uniform in the way we assess children with movement difficulties we will probably find that the factors become more stable.

In the clinical and educational world, more qualitative judgments can be made. For example, we often see children for whom handwriting presents a major problem. Computers, tablets and phones will continue to be used more widely but as organizations like the National Handwriting Association point out, handwriting is still a major activity in both school and the workplace and slow and or illegible handwriting is a hindrance to success. Other children will have different specific difficulties, such as bicycle riding and general agility, hindering their participation in social activities. Rather than having specific difficulties there is also a group of children who have moderate overall problems and this general lack of skill has effects across the curriculum and in other areas of daily living. Decisions about therapy are made surrounding the importance of the profiles. A child with more general difficulties will require a different approach to one whose difficulties lie in one of two specific areas, such as handwriting or riding a bicycle, with decisions made by the child and relevant stakeholders.

## Summary

Movement is an integral part of daily life and most children achieve the skills necessary for daily life with some ease and apparently little thought. However, there are some for whom these activities are a constant challenge and often are a source of concern to the child and those close to them. A proportion of these children have poorly developed movement skills as a primary part of a diagnosis, and the major diagnostic condition for these children is DCD. For others, they will have an alternative diagnostic condition, but also show movement difficulties as a co-occurring problem. This is often the case in those diagnosed with disorders such as dyslexia, ADHD, ASD and DLD. Research shows that without intervention, most of these children have problems that stay with them as they enter adolescence and indeed adulthood. For all these children, in most cases, some form of intervention and support is considered desirable. In the following chapters we will look at the principles of this support through to the intervention and support processes.

We list below the key features of the importance of competent movement across the developmental continuum. The listing is not necessarily in order of importance but captures all the important considerations in both evaluating and constructing effective interventions for those individuals who fall under the different diagnostic descriptions.

- Movement is the only way we interact with both others and our environment.

- Most children develop appropriate movement skills.

- A number have a movement difficulty with a primary movement diagnostic condition, such as DCD.

- Others, such as those with ADHD, DLD, ASD and dyslexia will show a higher prevalence of movement difficulties than typically developing peers.

- Children with movement difficulties show effects in daily living in both movement and other contexts.

- DSM-5 details all the above developmental disorders.

- Causes of the movement difficulties are variable and often unknown.

- Prevalence rates in DCD vary', but around 5% will require immediate attention and up to 15% will require monitoring for progress.

- Sex differences are evident.

## References

APA (2000) *Diagnostic and Statistical Manual of Mental Disorders,* 4th edition, Text Revision (DSM-IV). Washington, DC: American Psychiatric Association.

APA (2013*) Diagnostic and Statistical Manual of Mental Disorders*, 5th Edition (DSM-5). Washington, DC: American Psychiatric Association.

Asperger H (1944) Autistic pathology in childhood. Translated and annotated In: Frith U (1991) *Autism and Asperger syndrome.* New York: Cambridge University Press, pp. 37–92.

Ayres JR (1979) *Sensory Integration and the Child.* Los Angeles, CA: Western Psychological Services.

Barkley RA (1997) Behavioural inhibition, sustained attention and executive functions: constructing a unifying theory of ADHD. *Psychol Bull* 121: 65–94.

Baron-Cohen S, Leslie A, Frith U (1985) Does the autistic child have a 'theory of mind'? *Cognition* 21: 37–46.

Baron-Cohen S (2008) Theories of the autistic mind. *The Psychologist,* 21, 2: 112–116.

Baron-Cohen S (2010) Empathising and systemising and the extreme male brain theory of autism. *Prog Brain Res* 186: 167–175.

Bishop DVM (2002) The role of genes in the etiology of specific language impairment. *J Commun Dis* 35: 311–328.

Bishop DVM (2007) Curing dyslexia and attention deficit hyperactivity disorder by training motor coordination: miracle or myth? *J Paediatr Child Health* 43: 653–655.

Blank R, Smits-Engelsman B, Polatajko H, Wilson P (2012) European Academy for Childhood Disability (EACD): recommendations on the definition, diagnosis and intervention of developmental coordination disorder (long version). *Dev Med Child Neurol* 54: 54–93.

Blank R, Barnett AL, Cairney J, et al. (2019) International clinical practice recommendations on the definition, diagnosis, assessment, intervention, and psychosocial aspects of developmental coordination disorder. *Dev Med Child Neurol* 61: 242–285.

Bornstein MH, Hahn C-S, Suwalsky JTD (2013) Physically developed and exploratory young infants contribute to their own long-term academic achievement. *Psychol Sci* 24: 1906–1917.

Bruininks RH (1978) *Bruininks-Oseretsky Test of Motor Proficiency*. Circle Pines MN: American Guidance Service.

Cacola P, Miller H, Williamson P (2107) Behavioral comparisons in autistic spectrum disorder and developmental coordination disorder: A systematic literature review. *Res Autistm Spectr Disord* 38: 6–18.

Campos JJ, Anderson DI, Barbu-Roth MA, Hubbard EM, Hertenstein MJ, Witherington D (2000) Travelling Broadens the Mind. *Infancy* 2: 149–219.

Cantell MH, Smyth MM, Ahonen TP (1994) Clumsiness in adolescence: educational, motor and social outcomes of motor delay detected at 5 years. *Adapt Phys Act Q* 1: 61–63.

Cantell M, Smyth MM, Ahonen TP (2003) Two distinct pathways for developmental coordination disorder: persistence and resolution. *Hum Move Sci* 22: 413–431.

Cantin N, Polatajko HJ, Thach WT, Jaglal S (2007) Developmental coordination disorder: Exploration of a cerebellar hypothesis. *Hum Mov Sci* 26: 491–509.

Cope N, Harold D, Moskvina V, et al. (2005) Strong evidence that KIAA0319 on chromosome 6p is a susceptibility gene for developmental dysfunction. *Am J Hum Gene* 4: 581–591.

Davids K, Button C, Bennett S (2008) *Dynamics of Skill Acquisition: A Constraints-led Approach*. Champaign Illinois: Human Kinetics.

DeFries JC, Alarcon M (1996) Genetics of specific reading disability. *Ment Retard Dev Dis Res Rev* 2: 39–47.

Denkla MB (1974) Development of motor coordination in normal children. *Dev Med Child Neurol* 16: 729–741.

Elliott JG, Grigorenko EL (2014) *The Dyslexia Debate*. Cambridge: Cambridge University Press.

Fawcett AJ, Nicholson RI (1995) Persistent deficits in motor skill acquisition of children with dyslexia. *J Mot Behav* 27: 235–240.

Fawcett AJ, Nicholson RI (1999) Performance of dyslexic children on cerebellar and cognitive tasks. *J Mot Behav* 31: 68–78.

Fleishman EA (1964) *The Structure and Measurement of Physical Fitness*. Englewood Cliffs, New Jersey: Prentice Hall.

Frith U (2003) Autism: *Explaining the Enigma*, 2nd edition. Oxford: Blackwell.

Gaines R, Collins D, Boycott K, Missiuna C, de Laat D, Soucie H (2008). Clinical expression of developmental coordination disorder in a large Canadian family. *Pediatr Child Health* 9: 763–768.

Geuze RHG (2017) On constraints and affordances in motor development and learning-the case of developmental coordination disorder. A commentary on Wade and Kuzek. *Hum Mov Sci* 57: 505–509.

Gillberg C, Kadesjo B (2003) Why bother about clumsiness? The implications of having developmental coordination disorder (DCD). *Neural Plast* 10: 59–68.

Green D, Baird G, Barnett AL, Henderson L, Huber J, Henderson SE (2002) The severity of motor impairment in Asperger's Syndrome: a comparison with specific developmental disorder of motor function. *J Child Psychol Psychiatry* 43: 655–668.

Green D, Baird G (2005) DCD and overlapping conditions. In: Sugden DA Chambers ME (eds). *Children with Developmental Coordination Disorder,* London: Whurr, pp. 93–118.

Green D, Charman T, Pickles A, et al. (2009) Impairment of movement skills of children with autistic spectrum disorders. *Dev Med Child Neurol* 51: 311–316.

Gubbay SS (1975) *The Clumsy Child*. London: Saunders.

Hadders-Algra M (2003) Developmental coordination: is clumsy motor behaviour caused by a lesion of the brain at an early age. *Neural Plast* 10: 39–50.

Hallet M, Lebiedowska MK, Thomas SL, Stanhope SJ, Denkla MB Rumsey J (1993) Locomotion of autistic adults. *Arch Neurol* 50: 1304–1308.

Harold D, Paracchini S, Scerri T, et al. (2006) Further evidence that the KIAA0319 gene confers susceptibility to developmental dyslexia. *Mol Psychiatry* 11: 1085–1091.

Henderson SE, Sugden DA (1992) *Movement Assessment Battery for Children: Manual* Sidcup: Psychological Corporation, p. 240.

Henderson SE, Sugden DA, Barnett A (2007) *Movement Assessment Battery for Children-2, Kit and Manual*. London: Harcourt Assessment, p. 194.

Hill EL (1998) A dyspraxic deficit in specific language impairment and developmental coordination disorder? Evidence from hand and arm movements. *Dev Med Child Neurol* 40: 388–395.

Hill EL (2001) Non-specific nature of specific language impairment: a review of the literature with regard to concomitant motor impairments. *Int J Lang Commun Disord* 36: 149–171.

Hill EL (2004) Executive function in autism. *Trends Cog Sci* 8: 26–32.

Hoare D (1994) Subtypes of developmental coordination disorder. *Adapt Phys Activ Q* 11: 158–169.

Hulme C, Snowling MJ (2009) *Developmental Disorders of Language Learning and Cognition*. Chichester: Wiley-Blackwell.

Iversen S, Berg K, Ellertsen B, Tønnessen FE (2005) Motor coordination difficulties in a municipality group and in a clinical sample of poor readers. *Dyslexia* 11: 217–231.

Iverson JM (2010) Developing language in a developing body: the relationship between motor development and language development. *J Child Lang* 37: 229–261.

Jansiewicz EM, Goldberg MC, Newscaffer CJ, Denkla MB, Landa R, Mostofsky SH (2006) Motor signs distinguish children with high functioning autism and Asperger's Syndrome from controls. *J Autism Dev Disord* 36: 613–621.

Johnson CJ, Beitchman JH (2006) Specific developmental disorders of speech and language. In: Gillberg C, Harrington R, Steinhausen H (eds) *A Clinician's Handbook of Child and Adolescent Psychiatry*. Cambridge, UK: Cambridge University Press.

Kadesjo B, Gillberg C (1999) Attention deficits and clumsiness in Swedish 7-year-old children. *Dev Med Child Neurol* 40: 796–804.

Kagerer FA, Contreras-Vidal JL, Bo J, Clarke JE (2006) Abrupt, but not gradual visuomotor distortion facilitates adaptation in children with developmental coordination disorder. *Hum Mov Sci* 25: 622–633.

Kaiser ML, Schoemaker MM, Albaret JM, Geuze RH (2015) What is the evidence of impaired motor skills and motor control among children with attention deficit hyperactivity disorder (ADHD)? Systematic review of the literature. *Res Dev Disabil* 36: 338–357.

Kanner L (1943) Autistic disturbances of affective contact. *Nerv Child* 2: 217–250.

Kaplan B, Crawford S, Wilson B, et al. (1997) Comorbidity of developmental coordination disorder and different types of reading disability. *J Int Neuropsych Soc* 3: 54.

Kaplan BJ, Crawford S, Cantell M, Kooistra L, Dewey D (2006) Comorbidity co-occurrence continuum: what's in a name? *Child Care Health Dev* 32: 723–731.

Kaplan BJ, Crawford SG, Wilson N, Dewey DM (1998) Comorbidity of developmental coordination disorder and different types of reading disability. *J Int Neuropsychol Soc* 3: 54.

Kaplan BJ, Wilson BN, Dewey DM, Crawford SG (1998) DCD may not be a discrete disorder. *Hum Mov Sci* 17: 471–490.

Kirby A, Sugden DA, Beveridge SE, Edwards L, Edwards R (2008a) Dyslexia and developmental coordination disorder in further and higher education. *Dyslexia* 3: 197–213.

Kirby A, Sugden DA, Beveridge SE, Edwards L (2008b) Developmental coordination disorder and adolescents and adults in further and higher education. *J Res Spec Educ Needs* 3: 120–131.

Kirby A, Edwards L, Sugden DA, Rosenbaum S (2010) The development and standardization of the Adult Developmental Co-ordination Disorders/Dyspraxia Checklist (ADC). *Res Dev Disabil* 1: 131–139.

Kirby A, Edwards L, Sugden DA (2011) Emerging adulthood in developmental coordination disorder: parent and young adult perspectives. *Res Dev Disabil* 32: 1351–1360.

Kita Y, Suzuki K, Hirata S, Sakihara K, Inagaki M, Nakai A (2016) Applicability of movement assessment battery for children, second edition to Japanese children: a study of age band 2. *Brain Dev* 38: 706–713.

Lingam R, Hunt L, Golding J, Jongmans M, Emond A (2009) Prevalence of developmental coordination disorder using the DSM-IV at 7 years of age: a popluation based study. *Pediatrics* 123: e693–e700.

Losse AM, Henderson SE, Elliman D, Hall D, Knight E, Jongmans M (1991) Clumsiness in children: do they grow out of it? A ten year follow-up. *Dev Med Child Neurol* 33: 55–68.

Macnab JJ, Miller LT, Polatajko HJ (2001) The search for subtypes in DCD: is cluster analysis the answer? *Hum Mov Sci* 20: 49–72.

Missiuna C, Gaines R, McLean J, de Laat D, Egan M, Soucie H (2007) Description of children identified by physicians as having developmental coordination disorder. *Dev Med Child Neurol* 11: 839–844.

Miyahara M (1994) Subtypes of students with learning disabilities based upon gross motor functions. *Adapt Phys Activ Q* 11: 368–383.

Mon-Williams MA, Wann JP, Pascal E (1999) Visual-proprioceptive mapping in children with developmental coordination disorder. *Dev Med Child Neurol* 41: 247–254.

Morton J (2004) *Understanding Developmental Disorders*. Oxford: Blackwell.

Mostofsky SH, Dubey P, Jerath VK, Jansiewicz EM, Goldberg MC, Denkla MB (2006) Developmental dyspraxia is not limited to imitation in children with autistic spectrum disorders. *J Int Neuropsychol Soc* 12: 314–326.

Mostofsky SH, Burgess P, Gidley Larson JC (2007) Increased motor cortex white matter volume predicts motor impairment in autism. *Brain* 130: 2117–2122.

Mostofsky SH, Powell SK, Simmonds DJ, Goldberg MC, Caffo B, Pekar JJ (2009) Decreased connectivity and cerebellar activity in autism during motor task performance. *Brain* 132: 2413–2425.

Mottron L, Belleville S, Rouleau G, Collignon O (2014) Linking neocortical, cognitive and genetic variability in autism with alterations of brain plasticity. 47: 735–752.

Newell KM (1986) Development of coordination. In: Wade MG, Whiting HTA (eds). *Motor Development in Children: Aspects of Coordination and Control.* Dordrecht: Martinus Nijhoff, pp. 341–360.

Newell KM, Scully P, Baillargeon R (1989) Task constraints and infant grip configuration. *Dev Psychobiol* 22: 817–832.

Nicolson R, Fawcett A, Dean P (2001) Developmental dyslexia: the cerebellar hypothesis. *Trends Neurosci* 24: 508–511.

Noterdaeme M, Mildenberger K, Minow F, Amorosa H (2002). Evaluation of neuromotor deficits in children with autism and children with a specific speech and language deficit. *Eur J Adolesc Psychiatry* 11: 219–225.

Orton ST (1937) *Reading, Writing and Speech Problems in Children.* New York: WW Norton and Co.

Pereira H, Eliasson A-C, Forssberg H (2000) Detrimental control of precision grip lifts in children with ADHD. *Dev Med Child Neurol* 42: 545–553.

Piek JP (2003) The role of variability in early infant motor development. *Infant Behav Dev* 25: 452–465.

Piek JP, Bradbury GS, Elsley SC, Tate T (2008) Motor coordination and social emotional behaviour in pre school-aged children. *Int J Disabil Dev Educ* 55: 143–152.

Powell RP, Bishop DVM (1992) Clumsiness and perceptual problems in children with specific language impairment. *Dev Med Child Neurol* 34: 755–765.

Ramussen P, Gillberg C (200) Natural outcome of ADHD with developmental coordination disorder at age 22 years: a controlled longitudinal community- based study. *J Am Child Adolesc Psychiatry* 39: 1424–1431.

Rarick GL, Dobbins DA, Broadhead GD (1976) *The Motor Domain and its Correlates in Educationally Handicapped Children.* Englewood Cliffs, NJ: Prentice Hall.

Rivard L, Missiuna C, Mc Cauley D, Cairney J (2014) Descriptive and factor analysis of DCDQ in a population-based sample of children with and without developmental coordination disorder. *Child, Care, Health Dev* 1: 42–49.

Rogers SJ, Benetto L, McEvoy R Pennington BF (1996) Inmitation and pantomine in high functioning adolescents with autistic spectrum disorders. *Child Dev* 6: 2060–2073.

Rutter M, Maughan B (2002) School effectiveness findings 1979-2002. *J Sch Psychol* 40: 451–475.

Rutter M, Yule W (1975) The concept of specific reading retardation. *J Child Psychiatry Psychol* 16: 18–197.

Schultz J, Henderson SE, Sugden DA, Barnet AL (2011) Structural validity of the Movement ABC Test: factor structure comparisons across three age groups. *Res Dev Disabil* 32: 1361–1369.

Sinani C, Sugden DA, Hill EL (2011) Gesture production in school vs clinical samples of children with developmental coordination disorder (DCD) and typically developing children (TDC). *Res Dev Disord* 32: 127–182.

Skinner RA, Piek JP (2001) Pscholsocial implications of poor motor coordination in chidlren and adolescents. *Hum Mov Sci* 20: 73–94.

Smith L, Gasser M (2005) The development of embodied cognition: six lessons from babies. *Artif Life* 11: 13–29.

Sugden DA (2017) Developmental Coordination Disorder: the road less travelled. *Hum Mov Sci* 57: 501–504.

Sugden DA, Wade MG (2013) *Typical and Atypical Motor Development*. Clinics in Developmental Medicine. London: Mac Keith Press.

Sugden DA, Wright H (1998) *Motor Coordination Disorders in Children*. Thousand Oaks, CA: Sage Publishers, p. 131.

Sugden DA, Wright HC (1996) The nature of developmental coordination disorder: inter and intra group differences. *Adapt Phys Activ Q* 13: 358–374.

Teitelbaum P, Teitelbaum O, Nye JM, Fryman J, Maurer RG (1998) Movement analysis in infancy may be useful for early diagnosis of autism. *Proc Natl Acad Sci USA* 95: 13982–13987.

Tseng MH, Henderson A, Chow SMK, Yao G (2004) Relationship between motor proficiency, attention, impulse and activity in children with ADHD. *Dev Med Child Neurol* 46: 381–388.

Visser J (2007) Subtypes and comorbidity in developmental coordination disorder. In: RH Geuze (ed.). *Developmental Coordination Disorder: A Review of Current Approaches.* Marseilles: Solal, pp. 9–25.

Wade MG, Kazek M (2017) Developmental coordination disorder and its cause: The road less travelled. *Hum Mov Sci* 57: 489–500.

Wade MG (2018) Mostly old wines in new bottles. Reply to commentaries. *Hum Mov Sci* 58: 16–24.

Wilson PH, Caeyenberghs K, Dewey D, Smits-Engelsman B, Steenbergen B (2018) Hybrid is not a dirty word: Commentary on Wade and Kazeck (2017). *Hum Mov Sci* 57: 510–515.

Wilson PH, Maruff P, Butson M, Williams J, Lum J, Thomas PR (2004) Impairments in the internal representation of movement in children developmental coordination disorder (DCD): a mental rotation task. *Dev Med Child Neurol* 46: 754–759.

Wilson PH, Ruddock S, Smits-Engelsman B, Polatajko H, Blank R (2013) Understanding performance deficits in developmental coordination disorder: a meta-analysis of recent research *Dev Med Child Neurol* 55: 217–228.

Wilson PH (2014) Neurocognitive processing deficits in children with DCD. In: Cairney J (ed.). *Developmental Coordination Disorder in Children: Consequences and Concurrent Problems.* Toronto: University of Toronto Press.

Wolpert DM, Doya K, Kawato M (2003) A unifying computational framework for motor control and social interaction. *Phil Trans Royal Soc* 358: 593–602.

World Health Organization (1992) *International Statistical Classification of Diseases and Related Health Problems*, 10th edition. Vol. 1. Geneva: World Health Organization.

Wright HC, Sugden DA (1996) A two-step procedure for the identification of children with developmental coordination disorder in Singapore. *Dev Med Child Neurol* 38: 1099–1106.

Yap RL, van der Leij A (1994) Testing the automatization deficit hypothesis of dyslexia via a dual task paradigm. *J Learn Disabil* 27: 660–665.

Zwicker JG, Missiuna C, Maled LA (2009) Neural correlates of developmental coordination disorder. *J Child Neurol* 24: 1273–1281.

Zwicker JG, Missiuna C, Harris SR, Boyd LA (2010) Brain activation of children with developmental coordination disorder is different than peers. *Pediatrics* 126: 678–686.

# Chapter 2

## Principles from motor learning

### Introduction

Movement, and its associated skill demands, is a common feature of the behaviour of all individuals, young and old, typical and atypical. In an earlier text we laid out in considerable detail the developmental trajectory of motor development for both typical and atypical children (Sugden and Wade 2013).

In this chapter we focus on the variables that mediate the acquisition of a range of motor skills, which either enhance or constrain recreational and sport related activities as well as many activities of daily living (ADL). We will not dwell on the possible underlying cause of deficits in learning motor skills, but emphasize the variables and protocols that research has identified as critical for the promotion of skill acquisition and, more importantly, lead to a relatively permanent change in performance.

As a starting point, we need to understand how an individual addresses the challenge of solving a motor problem? This can be a child's desire to copy an observed motor behaviour in order to engage in a play related activity. The likely next step would be to engage in self-directed trial and error activity in an attempt to 'copy' what is being observed. This approach may lead to some level of success but, according to the extant research into motor learning, a desired skill can be more rapidly acquired by employing evidence-based protocols on skill learning.

---

**Box 2.1** Skill classifications: discrete, serial and continuous

**Discrete skill**

A skilled action that requires a single act (e.g. switching a light on or off).

**Serial skill**

A series of single discrete activities produces a finished product, such as an automobile assembly line. In or in gymnastics a round-off or back somersault.

**Continuous skill**

A continuous skill is one that appears not to have an identifiable beginning or end-point, such as walking or swimming; other continuous activities are writing, riding a bicycle and skating.

Of the three classifications continuous skills seem less subject to forgetting.

---

## Skill classifications

Any action that requires accuracy or precision may be regarded as a skill. Yet all skills vary as to the parts of the body used, the complexity of the action (level of coordination required) and the temporal organization involved. Accordingly, it can be helpful to use a classification system to differentiate the rich variety of skillful activities. A relatively simple yet effective way to classify types of skilled activities is to separate them into *discrete, serial and continuous* skills. An alternative classification is that of *open* and *closed* skills. These are described in Box 2.1.

*Open and closed skills*

Open and closed skills relate to the environmental context in which the skill is being performed. In an enclosed arena where weather and surface are essentially constant. A free throw basketball shot would be classified as a *closed* skill as the court dimensions, ball size and hoop dimensions are all constant. In contrast an *open skill* might be playing tennis on an outdoor court where the players would have to contend with a court surface that may be wet or dry, wind conditions, and possibly the angle of the sun, all of which would require adjustments by the player in how to strike the ball and how to receive shots from the opponent. This situation has low predictability. In a *closed* skill setting the performer can exercise a higher degree of control simply because there is less variability as to the demands of the skill. In an *open* setting the individuals are subject to variations that are beyond their control, yet these variables influence the quality of the skilled action.

Gentile (1972) proposed a more detailed set of skill classifications with a finer-grained taxonomy of skilled activities, an example of which is presented below in Table 2.1.

**Table 2.1** Adapted format of Gentile's (1972) taxonomy of motor skills

| Environmental Context ↓ | Body Stability | | Body Movement | |
| --- | --- | --- | --- | --- |
| | No Object Manipulation | Object Manipulation | No Object Manipulation | Object Manipulation |
| Stationary regulatory condition and no-interval variability | 1a Practicing a golf swing without a club | 1b Hitting balls at a driving range from the same spot | 1c Practicing the same dance steps | 1d Practicing the same dance steps with a partner |
| Stationary regulatory condition and interval variability | 2a Practicing separate Tai Chi moves standing on the same spot | 2b Hitting ball with a cue from different locatinos on a billiards table | 2c Practicing different dance steps on own | 2d Practicing different dance steps with a partner |
| In-motion regulatory condition and no-interval variability | 3a Riding on a stationary exercise bike at a constant speed | 3b Fishing while sitting on a boat and only casting once | 3c Practicing lawn bowls delivery with a walking step without a bell | 3d Returning a tennis serve from a tennis ball pitching machine |
| In-motion regulatory condition and interval variability | 4a Riding on a stationary exercise bike at different speeds | 4b Fishing while standing on a boat; throwing cast out in a new spot each attempt | 4c Walking in a busy shopping centre | 4d Riding a bike on a bike path |

Gentile's classification describes in more detail the relationships between the components of a skill. The central aim of her taxonomy was to provide a functional guide for therapists and coaches to assist in determining where a movement problem might reside and thus generate an appropriate intervention to address a specific skill-related deficit. As can be seen from Table 2.1, the taxonomy comprises a 4 × 4 matrix that depicts skilled activities as *stationary* vs *in-motion*, *object manipulation* vs *no manipulation* and *inter-trial variability* vs *no inter-trial variability*. Picking up or grasping a cup or throwing a dart at a target represent a *stationary environmental* context. Stepping onto a moving escalator or catching a baseball represent an *in-motion environmental* context. Employing Gentile's taxonomy in order to evaluate an individual's movement capabilities might proceed as follows:

1. Stand unassisted (category 1A).

2. Stand unassisted holding an object (category 1B).

3. Walk a specified distance in an uncluttered pathway (category 1C).

4. Walk a specified distance while holding a coffee cup (category 1D).

From this starting point, other elements of the taxonomy can be introduced, depending on the specific goals of the therapist and the individual client's needs. It should be remembered that Gentile's taxonomy was developed for typically developed adults. Other considerations would be required when applying this taxonomy to children or adults with special needs. However, there would certainly be the tendency for such individuals to exhibit a higher level of performance variability, and in some cases, a slower rate of reaching an acceptable level of performance criterion.

## Performance versus learning: is there a difference?

*Performance* in a motor skill is the temporary outcome of a particular attempt at a task. This may be a golf shot that is particularly good, rolling a piece of pastry into the shape, or sawing a particularly difficult piece of wood. It is not a permanent change in behaviour as it could alter when the individual tries to do it again. *Learning*, on the other hand, in any context, implies a relatively permanent change in behaviour. Thus, learning cannot be 'seen', it can only be inferred from what is observed, and that is what is termed 'performance'. Accordingly, as we practice a skilled activity, we can observe an increase in our level of performance, whether achieved by self-directed trial and error or through the benefits of an instructor. To determine if learning has actually occurred as a result of this practice, a true test is to determine if this increase or improvement is permanent. How is 'permanent change' measured? To record some level of permanent change we use *a retention test* to determine if the performance is 'somewhat permanent' and to see if there is any appreciable decay between the end of practice period and recording the level of performance after a break. If an individual produces a level of performance close to what was achieved at the end of the practice period, this is evidence that learning has taken place. If this is the case, we can conclude that a 'somewhat permanent change' has occurred and learning has taken place.

The challenge in teaching individuals to improve their motor skills is to determine the best way to structure the practice sessions and what kinds of feedback to provide the learner. A substantial amount of empirical research has been focused on the learning of motor skills. The difference between performance and learning is important for teaching children with movement difficulties. Any single level of performance may not measure learning (i.e. how permanent the performance level is) and so we must look at some of the more substantial and relatively permanent outcomes to determine if learning has taken place. Some of these possible 'outcomes' are listed below. Learning is measured by observing multiple performances over time and can involve any or a combination of the following:

- **Improvement/accomplishment in performance**
  The child can now perform a skill or perform it better than previously.

  A young person with developmental coordination disorder (DCD) can now ride a bicycle and engage with peers.

  A child with cerebral palsy (CP) can successfully reach and pick up an object not previously possible.

  A child with DCD can now write so that others can read it.

- **Consistency and stability in performance**
  A child with CP can now pick up an object 80% of the time as opposed to 40% previously.

  Children with DCD can now dress themselves quickly enough so that they are not embarrassed in physical education lessons.

  A child who had difficulty selecting what to attend to can now focus on the main part of the motor task, enabling them to practice appropriately.

- **More adaptable performance**
  A child with CP can reach for different shaped cups in school, at home and in friends' houses, or can reach around other obstacles to grasp a cup.

  Children with attention-deficit–hyperactivity disorder (ADHD) can give more sustained attention to a novel motor task.

  A child with autism spectrum disorder (ASD) can interact and cooperate with another child on their chosen motor task.

- **Transitioning from part-task to whole-task performance**
  Reaching and grasping by a child with CP no longer requires two distinct movements of reach and then grasp, but is all achieved in one action.

  A child with DCD can now throw while 'on the run' and does not have to stop to make it two movements.

- **Performance becomes more automatic, shown by being able to do two things at once**
  The child with CP can now argue with her brother as she reaches to pick up the cup.

  The child with a speech and language impairment can talk to a therapist at the same time as executing a movement.

- **Flexible use of freezing and freeing degrees of freedom**
  A child with CP can now exhibit greater movement flexibility, according to a specific context, such as pouring water from a full cup into an empty cup to make the water levels in each cup equal. This requires both 'freezing' and 'freeing' of degrees of freedom (DoF).

  A child can progress from learning to play a tune on a violin or other stringed instrument, constrained by a limited number of DoF, to being able play a more flexible set of tunes. This freezing and freeing of the DoF, according to task demands, could also apply to an activity such as learning to snow ski by first learning a 'snow plough' before moving on to a more flexible set of skiing activities. Similarly, a child with DCD can use a paintbrush or a pen or pencil without having to steady it with the other hand.

Before describing the specific variables and the associated research that has influenced the acquisition of motor skills, it should be noted that *any* learned skill occurs in the context of the relationship between the skill being learned, the resources possessed by the learner, and the environmental context wherein the learning takes place. We have referred to this in Chapter 1 as the Task-Performer and Environment (TPE) model (Newell 1986).

In the case of individuals who have additional constraints that are a consequence of diagnoses such as DCD, autistic spectrum disorder (ASD) and attention-deficit–hyper-activity disorder (ADHD), the challenge of learning a specific motor skill is likely to require strategies for the most efficient way to promote learning. The variables central to the acquisition of a motor skill comprise (1) the *type* or *classification* of skill to be learned; (2) the *structure* of the practice regimen to best facilitate learning; and (3) the most effective type of *instruction*, *demonstration* and *feedback* provided to the learner. All these factors must be considered within the context of each individual's specific diagnosis. It should be noted that much of the research on motor skill learning has been conducted primarily with university students, the majority of whom are typical rather than atypical in their developmental trajectory.

## How learning progresses

*Cognitive to associative to autonomous learning*
As we have already noted above, an individual who seeks to improve his or her performance of a particular skill usually adopts a trial and error methodology, i.e. the individual is left to his or her own devices to improve. Improvement may occur but, a more structured approach to practice typically yields a more efficient and faster rate of improvement.

Without delving too deeply into the theoretical aspects of skill learning, it will be helpful to view the process of acquiring a motor skill from the perspective advanced by Fitts and Posner (1967). Paul Fitts and Michael Posner were psychologists interested in human performance and in their 1967 paper proposed that in learning any skill, the individual progresses through three stages: (1) the *cognitive* stage, (2) the *associative* stage and (3) the *automaticity* stage. A good example of this process would be learning to operate a manual (stick shift) gear system in a car. Here the challenge is to first learn and understand the relationship between operating the clutch pedal and the accelerator (gas pedal) in such a way as to not stall the vehicle. At this *cognitive* stage of the task the learner must pay close attention to understanding the coordinated relationship between the clutch and the accelerator and the layout and design of the manual gearbox, but this leaves little time to focus on the actual direction of vehicle. Practicing this initial cognitive stage is best done in a large parking lot well away from traffic. After some practice the learner begins to acquire the necessary operational techniques of changing gears and not stalling the vehicle; this is the *associative* stage of learning. Finally, after further practice the *automaticity* stage is reached whereby the manipulation of the manual transmission and the operating of both the clutch and accelerator become second nature and the driver can pay full attention to driving the vehicle safely in traffic.

*Understanding comes through consistency to adaptability*
Other ways to look at this progression are provided by Gentile and other proponents of dynamical systems. Gentile (2000) describes two stages rather than three, with the first encompassing much of Fitts and Posner's first two stages and the second dealing with abilities such as adaptability and consistency. Again, instructions, explanations, demonstrations and feedback will vary according to where the individual is in the learning process. As stated by Gentile (2000), much depends on whether the individual is stationary or in motion; the context (is object manipulation required?) and so on.

*A constraints dynamical systems approach to learning*
A rather different way to look at the learning process is provided by those advocating a dynamical systems approach (Bernstein 1967; Whiting 1984). In this approach, learning progresses through a continuing attunement of the body to the environmental demands. The recruitment of coordinative structures (groups of muscles acting together) is softly

assemble, according to environmental demands. In the early stages of learning, fewer DoF will be used for a given task, progressing to more DoF being used as the child becomes more accomplished. This progression allows the child to adapt more efficiently to any changing environmental circumstances. The proponents describe it as involving a progression from the *freezing to the freeing and exploiting of the DoF*. For example, people learning to ski typically learn first the 'snow plough' a constrained activity (freezing DoF), which demonstrates how shifting weight to the right ski will produce a left turn of direction while shifting the weight to the left ski results in a right turn. While this may result in early, but limited, success for the beginner, it is far from the more flexible (freeing DoF) skiing that a more accomplished skier can demonstrate.

The teaching focus of many motor skills, whether sport related, ADL or similar activities, is first on limiting the DoF, which ensures some initial success. Having achieved initial success, progress towards a more flexible iteration of the skill is possible as the learner begins to 'free' the DoF.

As stated above, the basis of all skilled activity is the interaction between the performer, the task and the environment (Newell 1986). Depending on the type of skill, the actual performance trajectory can vary, as illustrated in the Figure 2.1.

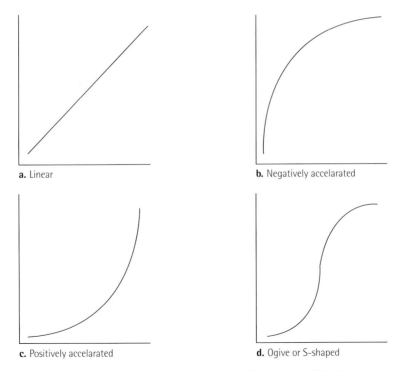

**a.** Linear

**b.** Negatively accelarated

**c.** Positively accelarated

**d.** Ogive or S-shaped

**Figure 2.1** Typical shapes of performance curves, depending on the skill being learned.

Different types of skill can produce different acquisition trajectories. Linear acquisition (Fig. 2.1a) shows a regular linear relationship between time in practice (horizontal scale) and rate of performance (vertical scale). For each unit of practice there is a corresponding increase in performance. Figure 2.1b depicts a relatively fast initial rate of acquisition then a slowing of improvement once the basics of the skill have been achieved. Figure 2.1c.shows just the opposite: a slower rate of acquiring the basic skill characteristics and then once acquired, a fairly rapid increase in performance. Figure 2.1d shows a mix of both the trajectories illustrated in parts 1b and1c, with an initial rapid increase in performance followed by a marked slowing of incremental performance increase at a higher level (an Ogive or S-shaped curve). This suggests something like a ceiling affect that requires a relatively greater amount of practice to bring about a small incremental improvement in performance. These four general types of performance curve illustrate the coordination properties of different skilled activities. An illustration of how an individual acquires a skill does not imply a theoretical basis as to how that skill is learned. All the illustrations in Figure 2.1 can be explained by both the current theoretical models of skill learning: information processing or the more recent dynamical systems theory. The focus here is less on any theoretical account for what is observed and more concerned with the practical aspects of how to structure effective practice for therapeutic interventions. As should be understood from the discussion so far, different kinds of skill require different ways of structuring the practice necessary to acquire or improve performance. We will now review how to structure practice for more effective learning.

## The structure of practice

The models we have described can all serve as good examples of how practice might be structured and scheduled to maximize the learning process. Here we discuss three important and well-known characteristics of practice, namely, massed versus distributed practice, block, serial or random practice and what is termed 'contextual interference'.

Practice alone does not always produce the desired or hoped for improvement in performance. Practice requires a more detailed focus on what elements are to be practiced and how to make such practice more efficient. Below we describe different methods of structuring practice and how a particular practice structure is best suited to a particular type of skill.

*Massed and distributed practice*
When practicing a skill, it is perhaps intuitive on the part of the instructor to allow the learner to have short rest periods distributed between bouts of practice trials so as not to fatigue the learner or avoid boredom or inattention. While this makes intuitive sense, the question is does one practice protocol show any advantage over the other? The question as to which is the better schedule of practice, massed versus distributed has resulted in the following conclusion: for continuous skills, such as swimming and riding a bicycle, it would seem that *distributed* practice is the most desirable; for discrete skills a *massed* practice

schedule (i.e. practicing without rest periods) may produce the best results. Clearly there are caveats as to which form of practice is best. Again, much will depend on the actual task and also the environmental context in which the skill is to be learned and executed.

Finally, for the purposes of this book, the status and abilities of a child with special needs must be taken into account. It should be remembered that almost all the published empirical research on motor behaviour was conducted using samples of university undergraduates, who represent a specific subset of the population at large. When applying the principles of motor learning discussed in this chapter to children who have a range of both motor and behavioural challenges, one should proceed with caution and recognize that specific clinical populations may not respond in the same way as suggested by the extant research. For example, reaction time and movement time in typical individuals are slower and more variable. In sport, a typical adult can capitalize on the limits an individual has to react (reaction time in adults is approximately 200msecs). For example, a rugby player may signal he or she plans to move to the right of a defender by 'faking' such a move; once committed the defender cannot start or stop that incorrect motion in less than an 200msecs, and that is before he or she starts to respond by moving. By that time the runner has moved past the defender by moving left. In a similar fashion a tennis player may appear to be hitting a forehand return, but in fact hits to the opponents backhand. The opponent again moves to play a forehand return and is wrong footed by being unable to start to change direction in less than the reaction time (200msecs). In both these examples the movement time is an additional variable.

### The structure of practice: blocked, serial and random

When introducing scheduled practice of a new skill the instructor is faced with a variety of ways to organize practice session. Intuitively, an instructor might reason that learning requires steady and focused practice to acquire the skill level that is the goal. In many cases, a specific skill has to be performed in a variety of situations or contexts. For example, learning to walk again after knee or hip replacement surgery requires the patient to walk on a level surface, up or down stairs and in situations where the surface may vary. Accordingly, any practice schedule needs to take into account circumstances that may require the skill to be executed in a variety of situations. Thus, a patient learning to walk after knee surgery might have three separate practice scenarios: walking on a flat smooth surface, walking on an uneven surface and ascending or descending a stairs. The instructor or therapist must decide how best to structure a practice schedule that will provide the maximum return with respect to learning (or relearning in this case) the skill.

Logic might dictate that it would be best to start with walking on a smooth surface, reasoning that once learned the person could move on to the next situation, i.e. walking on an uneven surface. Once that has been achieved he or she can move on to the stair-climbing task. But what does the research tell us about this scenario?

Again, we must remember that the performance level reached after a series of practice trials does not reliably indicate the level of learning. Learning is a *relatively* permanent change in performance, and performance recorded at the end of a series of practice trials may not represent a permanent change. Measuring the level of performance after a break in the practice regimen is a reliable way to determine if the performance gain is permanent. This is referred to as a *retention* test. The research that shows how best to achieve a permanent change in performance considers the best order to schedule practice on the skill to be learned and the various situations where the skill needs to be executed. As noted above, these can be blocked practice, serial practice or random practice (Table 2.2).

We have described the intuitive, and some say logical, approach, which is blocked practice: practicing each of the three separate skills and reaching an acceptable level of performance in the first skill before moving to the next. However, research on the structure of practice suggests a different approach.

In any skill-learning setting it is desirable that the individual be engaged in the learning process and it is the role of the instructor to maximize this engagement. Psychologist Robert Bjork (1994) has coined the term 'desirable difficulties'. Bjork described these

**Table 2.2** A structured practice schedule for three types of tennis shot (forehand, backhand, and overhead). Practice sessions are blocked, serial or random, with each session lasting 30 minutes. All groups practice for six consecutive days. Note the blocked practice is always 30 minutes, while the serial and random sessions are 5 minutes per practice type (serial or random)

| | | Class Day | | | | | |
|---|---|---|---|---|---|---|---|
| Practice | Minutes | 1 | 2 | 3 | 4 | 5 | 6 |
| Blocked | 30 | Forehand | Forehand | Backhand | Backhand | Overhead | Overhead |
| Serial | 5 | Forehand | Forehand | Forehand | Forehand | Forehand | Forehand |
| | 5 | Backhand | Backhand | Backhand | Backhand | Backhand | Backhand |
| | 5 | Overhead | Overhead | Overhead | Overhead | Overhead | Overhead |
| | 5 | Forehand | Forehand | Forehand | Forehand | Forehand | Forehand |
| | 5 | Backhand | Backhand | Backhand | Backhand | Backhand | Backhand |
| | 5 | Overhead | Overhead | Overhead | Overhead | Overhead | Overhead |
| Random | 5 | Backhand | Forehand | Overhead | Forehand | Backhand | Overhead |
| | 5 | Forehand | Overhead | Forehand | Overhead | Forehand | Forehand |
| | 5 | Backhand | Overhead | Overhead | Overhead | Backhand | Overhead |
| | 5 | Overhead | Backhand | Backhand | Backhand | Overhead | Backhand |
| | 5 | Backhand | Forehand | Backhand | Forehand | Backhand | Backhand |
| | 5 | Forehand | Forehand | Overhead | Forehand | Forehand | Forehand |

difficulties as varying the conditions of practice, rather than keeping them constant or predictable; distributed practice rather than mass practice; and finally introducing 'contextual interference' into the practice schedule.

### Contextual interference

The concept of contextual interference was developed by William Battig (1979), whose primary research interest was in human memory. Battig suggested that individuals respond to situations of high or low interference with correspondingly high or low levels of elaborative and distinctive processing, which can require increased effort. These ideas were extended to research on motor learning by Shea and Morgan (1979), especially as it relates to the structure of practice. Contextual interference has influenced a wide range of learning from how to best teach content in schools and universities to learning to differentiate species of birds. The central idea behind contextual interference is that the more random the practice schedule of a task the greater the engagement of the learner. This is achieved by making the unexpected delivery of a practice variation that may frustrate the learner early in practice, but will eventually draw him or her deeper into the underlying features of the skill he or she is learning. The practice schedule is illustrated in Table 2.2.

Table 2.2 illustrates a 6-day practice plan using three different practice schedules (blocked, serial and random) for the purpose of teaching three different types of tennis shots (forehand, backhand and overhead). Each practice session lasts 30 minutes and is divided into 5-minute segments, except for the blocked practice. This ensures an equal amount of practice time for each variation of the practice structure for the skill.

The level of contextual interference will vary, depending on the practice structure, with a higher level of contextual interference producing an initial reduction in the level of performance. However, across the 6 days of practice the retention level will improve compared to the seemingly more 'sensible or logical' blocked practice schedule. The random structure engages the learner more deeply in practicing the skill. In regard to its application to individuals who have difficulties with skill learning, it would seem a balanced approach would be best, beginning with a blocked approach for the individual to achieve initial success, then introducing a serial practice schedule and later a random schedule as the learner progresses and gains confidence. This progression will produce first a low level of contextual interference (blocked practice) with a progression to a higher level of contextual interference (random practice). Such a progression should keep the learner motivated and enhance retention of the specific skill being learned.

The three scenarios illustrated in Table 2.2 can be applied to a variety of recreational skills or ADL, with a blocked schedule of practicing each scenario before going on to the next. This would be followed by a serial schedule where, (returning to the example of the patient with knee surgery), the learner practices a combination of the three walking scenarios in order, and a random schedule where each of the three versions of walking is presented in a random order that could not be anticipated by the learner.

The random presentation is the 'difficulty' element described by Bjork (1994), which challenges the learner and seemingly slows the rate of performance. This is likely to be caused by the initial frustration of dealing with unexpected variations. The 'desirable' component is that the random presentation requires the learner to contend with the unexpected (random) presentation order and this leads eventually to a more focused (engaged) effort in developing the processes of learning that can result in long-term retention, which is the goal of the practice. It is this random, sometimes frustrating, situation that reflects contextual interference. The influence of contextual interference assumes that the motivation of the learner is enhanced by the 'desirable difficulties' that challenge him or her (Bjork 1994). This cannot be said of individuals with special needs, however, as much will depend on their intrinsic motivation.

Atypical individuals might be unable, or perhaps less able, to respond to the inherent frustration that contextual interference places on them. As noted above, a modified practice protocol may require first blocked practice, followed by serial practice, and finally using random practice as a long-term objective to be included in any practice schedule.

## Feedback in motor learning

The concept of feedback is both broad and diverse. It can be visual, auditory, olfactory, or anything that provides added information about a situation can be regarded as feedback. When we talk about the role of feedback with respect to learning a motor skill it is necessary to focus more specifically on what feedback includes. Humans have a rich internal source of feedback that emanates from within their body; we refer to this as *intrinsic* feedback. Receiving information about a skilled performance from outside of the human body is referred to as *augmented* feedback, i.e. information over and above what we 'feel' from within our body. A brief expansion on these two forms of feedback follows.

### Intrinsic feedback
Intrinsic feedback is sensory information from the tactile, visual and proprioceptive organs (joint and muscle). The sensation of touch (haptics) emanates from the mechanore-ceptors in the skin, which are stimulated by temperature and deformation. Proprioceptors (present in the muscle-joint system) via muscle spindles are embedded in the actual muscle fibers. These muscle spindles detect changes in both length and contractile veloc-ity of the muscle as a function of flexion or extension of the joint complex involved. Golgi tendons (located near the tendon insertion of the muscle) detect changes in muscle tension or force. Finally, a range of joint receptors located in the joint capsule and ligaments provide additional information about changes in joint movement. This physiological and anatomical array of information is a direct consequence of both

muscle and joint action. Given that humans possess essentially hundreds of bones and thousands of muscles, taken together these sensory neurons provide the central nervous system with a rich source of information regarding the status of the joint-muscle system of the individual, whether at rest or in motion. Proprioceptive information available from these sources contributes to maintaining stable coordination of limbs and body segments in three ways.

First, the maintenance of postural control requires information from vision and joint receptors, along with a functioning central nervous system (cerebellum and basal ganglia). Any damage to these interacting and sometimes redundant sources of postural stability can lead to an inability to control upright stance. Second is the spatial-temporal capacity to couple limbs and limb segments. Third is adaptation to movements that represent non-preferred coordination patterns, for example writing with your non-preferred hand.

The role of proprioception and kinesthesia in motor control and learning, balance and posture, adaptability and coordination has been well established, both in the published research literature and in clinical practice. In instances where the proprioceptive systems are impaired, either by trauma, disease or more subtle developmental anomalies, these can contribute to both the performance and, probably, the acquisition of skills. In addition to intrinsic feedback, such as that available from the somatosensory, vestibular and visual systems, an additional source of information about performance and skill learning can come from *augmented* feedback provided by the instructor.

### Augmented feedback
Augmented feedback can take two forms: knowledge of results or knowledge of performance.

### Knowledge of results
Knowledge of results informs the learner of their performance in the form of either a descriptor or a metric of the accuracy of each trial response in a series of practice trials. This type of knowledge of results can be given as a verbal descriptor [e.g. 'That was very good'; 'Good'; 'OK'; or 'You missed'). It can also be given as numeric feedback (e.g. 'That was long, 2)'; (That was short, 3)', and so on]. The form of the knowledge of results can depend, in part, on the developmental stage of the learner. Children may better understand a verbal form of knowledge of results while adults may be able to better utilize numeric feedback. In addition, when to deliver the knowledge of results has been the subject of research. Should it be given immediately after the end of a practice trial, halfway into the inter-trial interval (rest), or just before the start of the next trial? The protocol as to when to provide knowledge of results is typically illustrated in Figure 2.2.

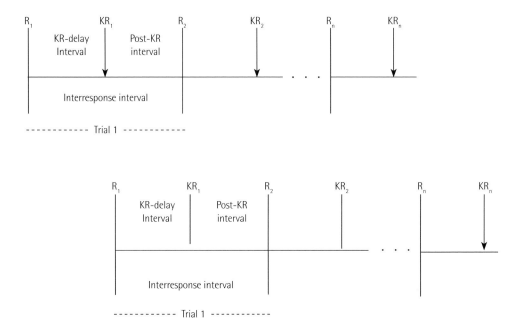

**Figure 2.2** Knowledge of result intervals for a trial to trial skill acquisition procedure. Imm, immediate; Del, delayed.

Figure 2.2 shows the periods between a series of trials in a hypothetical experiment where an individual performs a series of practice trials. During the rest interval between trials the experimenter can manipulate when to provide the knowledge of results of the just completed trial. The question surrounding the knowledge of results delay focuses on what activity the learner is engaging in during either the knowledge of results delay interval, or the post knowledge of results interval (see Fig. 2.3). The general consensus regarding the knowledge of results delay and the post-knowledge of results delay has produced mixed results as to the positive effects on the learner. The activities engaged in by the learner during these intervals can hinder, benefit or have no effect.

It is likely that much depends on the nature of the skill, the coordination required and the abilities of the learner. Again, much of the research data on this area has been gathered on typical university students. Disorders such as ADHD could have a serious impact on knowledge of results delay or post-knowledge of results delay. A final issue with respect to knowledge of results is how to best 'engage' the learner in the process of learning the selected skill. Typically, knowledge of results is provided after each trial in a series of trials, but research into the question of how often to inform the learner suggests that once the basic skill has been acquired there is value in delaying in some way the knowledge of results regarding the learner's responses. This may take the form

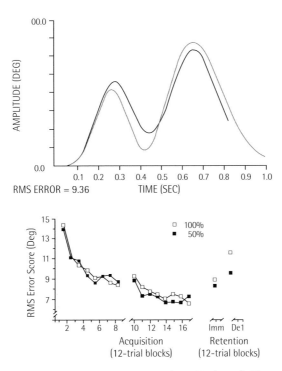

**Figure 2.3** This is an experiment by Winstein and Schmidt (1990). The top panel depicts the movement pattern superimposed on the target pattern. Note the target pattern lasts for 0.8 seconds. The bottom panel illustrates the results of the experiment when either 50% or 100% of knowledge of results is provided to the two groups of participants. Reprinted from Gentile AM (1972) by permission of the National Association for Kinesiology in Higher Education (NAKHE) www.nakhe.org.

of knowledge of results being given, for example, after a series of five trials, or providing summary knowledge of results after 10 trials.

To better illustrate this point, Figure 2.2a shows the results of a study by Winstein and Schmidt (1990), which asked participants to reproduce a particular pattern. Figure 2.2b shows the effect of providing both 100% knowledge of results and 50% knowledge of results. As can be observed in Figure 2.2b, both forms of knowledge of results had essentially the same effect during the acquisition trials; however during the immediate and delayed retention trials, the error scores for the 50% knowledge of results group were lower and more permanent than the 100% knowledge of results frequency.

This study suggests that a reduced frequency of knowledge of results may be beneficial for motor skill learning, but it may depend on the nature of the task to be learned. For our purposes it is important to recognize that the specific resources an atypical participant may or may not possess can have additional benefits or consequences on to how best to provide the frequency of knowledge of results in order to optimize learning.

Providing 100% feedback versus 50% feedback shows a clear advantage for the 50% condition in the retention test. The effects of providing some form of summary knowledge of results is clearly beneficial, once the learner has some level of familiarity with the skill to be learned. These two latter protocols appear to engage the learner more 'deeply' into understanding how best to develop the learning of the skill. Continuing to provide knowledge of results continuously after every trial may produce a situation where the learner is less focused on determining how to improve once the basic skill set has been acquired. Finally, knowledge of results has a motivational element in informing the learner of their progress. All of the techniques of delivering knowledge of results will depend on the nature of the skill, the developmental status of the individual learner and context in which the skill will both be learned and expressed.

### Knowledge of performance

Knowledge of performance refers to providing the learner with feedback that relates to the actual movement pattern (coordination) related characteristics of a performance; in other words, information about the actual coordination outcomes. An example might be the instructor telling the learner: ' Your left arm is not straight', showing a video of a performance and telling the learner what needs to be corrected with respect to the actual movements made as the skill is executed. Box 2.2 shows a contrast between knowledge of results and knowledge of performance.

---

**Box 2.2** Examples of either Knowledge of Performance (KP), or Knowledge of Results (KR) for a sport skill, or a rehabilitation session. Adapted from Magill and Anderson (2016).

| Diver | | |
|---|---|---|
| | KP KR | 'Watch the video and try to gain more height at take-off'. |
| | KP | 'See the judges score'. |
| Cricket stroke | | 'The video shows you are not following through with your stroke'. |
| | KR | 'Your shot was too high and you were caught out'. |
| Tennis serve | KP | 'Focus on completing your throw up'. |
| | KR | 'You threw the ball too close to yourself'. |
| Student driver in a simulator | KP | 'Try and keep the vehicle in the middle of your lane'. |
| | KR | 'Note the number of errors you made during practice'. |

Adapted from Magill and Anderson (2016).

As can be observed from Box 2.1, the nature of the instructor's comments depict either a knowledge of results form of feedback, usually related to some form of a metric, such as time or distance, and so on. The knowledge of performance feedback relates more to how the task was executed and the faults that might be observed via a video replay or what the instructor says with respect to form of the skill.

## Constraints on the performer

The central focus of this chapter is to consider the overall aspects of skill acquisition when atypical individuals are challenged to acquire a variety of motor skills and are constrained to some degree by a range of special needs. The bulk of the research described in this chapter has been compiled mostly on typically university students and as a result some of the 'take home messages' from this research will need to be carefully reviewed when applied to young people who have DCD, or some degree of ASD or ADHD. Nevertheless, the principles described in this chapter clearly influence the rate of skill acquisition and the long-term retention of those skills, and it should be noted that the long-term retention is indicative of learning. Performance acquired over a series of practice trials is not always retained in the long term.

The impact of physical growth and the associated consideration of body scale as it relates to perceptual–motor development must, of course, be considered. In a recent book Newell and Wade (2018) outline the theoretical framework of the ecological approach to perception and action and how changes in body scale and the timescale during growth clearly relate to the emergence and dissolution of the fundamental skills in infancy; and the perception of what the environment affords for action, together with the emergent pattern of movement coordination. These considerations apply equally to typical or atypical children with respect to their capacity to learn and retain motor skills.

The above principles provide a basis for developing training protocols for children with special needs, providing flexibility on the types of tasks and the structure of the practice sessions are at the forefront of the instructor or therapist's thinking.

## Summary

In this chapter we have focused on the variables that influence an individual acquiring a skilled activity in a more efficient manner. In addition to enhancing the rate of acquisition, research suggests that the rate of retention of the practiced activity will be enhanced and retained over a longer period of time. This is not to suggest that skills acquired will not require continued future practice, to retain what has been learned. Any skill that is either new or has to be relearned progresses in the context of the ongoing dynamic interrelationship between the task, the performer and the environment in which the learning and performance takes place. For the purposes of the book, the overriding consideration has been that the performer is likely to present with a range of special needs, all of which may present challenges to those charged with improving their quality of life.

## Notes to practitioners and clinicians

We understand that all practitioners, whether teachers, therapists or others, are faced with clients who present with a range of challenges. Accordingly, it is always valuable to keep in mind the following:

1. What we know about motor behaviour research is based largely on the results of studies. The participants in such research studies are typically university students, and not the clients you see in clinic.

2. The results of these laboratory studies do not always generalize to your clinical context, or the individuals for whom you are providing services.

3. While many clients will show slower response times and wider variability in their ability to acquire new skills, or re-learn past skills, rates of acquisition and the structure of any practice schedules will not strictly follow the research data from which such principles have been developed.

4. It is far more important to maintain levels of motivation and attention with clinical populations than the prior assumptions made when the related original research data was collected.

5. While you may deal with many of the known constraints of your clients, remember that much of the research on motor skills was collected in a laboratory setting, which may be a major constraint on the generalizability of the results when applied in real world clinical settings.

## References

Battig WF (1979) The flexibility of human memory. In: Cermak LS, Craik FIM (eds). *Levels of Processing in Human Memory* Hillsdale, NJ: Erlbaum, pp. 23–44.

Bernstein N (1967) *The Coordination and Regulation of Movements*. New York: Pergammon Press.

Bjork R (1994) Memory and meta-memory considerations in the training of human beings. In: Metcalfe, Shimamuru A. (eds). *Metacognition: Knowing about Knowing.* Cambridge, MA: MIT Press, pp. 185–205.

Brady F (2008) The contextual interference effect and sport skills. *Percept Mot Skills* 106: 461–472.

Fitts PM, Posner MI (1967) *Human Performance*. Belmont, CA: Brooks/Cole.

Gentile AM (1972) A working model of skill acquisition with application to teaching. *Quest* 17: 3–23.

Magill R, Anderson D (2016) *Levels of Motor Learning and Control: Concepts and Applications,* 11th Edition. New York: McGraw Hill.

Newell K, Wade M (2018) Physical growth, body scale, and perceptual-motor development. In: Plumert J (ed.). *Advances in Child Development and Behaviour,* Volume 55. Netherlands: Elsevier Press.

Shea JB, Morgan RL (1979) Contextual Interference effects on the acquisition, retention, and transfer of a motor skill. *J Exp Psychol Learn, Mem Cogn* 5: 179–187.

Shea CH, Kohl RM (1990) Specificity and variability of practice. *Res Q Exerc Sport* 62: 169–177.

Sugden DA, Wade MG (2013) *Typical and Atypical Motor Development.* Clinics in Developmental Medicine London: Mac Keith Press.

Thelen E (1995) Motor development: a new synthesis. *Am Psychol* 50: 79–95.

Turvey MT, Shaw RE, Mace W (1978) Issues in the theory of action: degrees of freedom, coordinative structures and coalitions. In: Requin J (ed.). *Perceiving, Acting and Knowing.* Hillsdale, NJ: Erlbaum, pp. 211–265.

Whiting HTA (1984) *Human Motor Actions: Bernstein Reassessed.* Amsterdam: North- Holland.

Winstein CJ, Schmidt RH (1990) Reduced frequency of knowledge of results enhances motor skill learning. *J Exp Psychol: Learn, Mem Cogn* 16: 677–691.

# Chapter 3

## Assessment and intervention

In this chapter, we introduce the concepts and activities of assessment and intervention, looking at generic aspects, what they are trying to achieve and some of the general principles that underpin the various approaches. Although later in the book we split the two activities of assessment and intervention into separate chapters, they do work together in a bidirectional manner so that assessment feeds into the intervention process, the results of which are relayed back and influence assessment practices.

Our *assessment procedures* are multiple, drawing upon observational and other data from parents, families and friends, and those in education and health settings. Our *intervention and support recommendations* arise from empirical studies based on sound theoretical foundations, together with clinical and other reports from professional key workers and families.

## Assessment and intervention working together

Our view has always been that although assessment and intervention are seen as separate entities, in reality and practice they are inextricably linked. An accurate assessment leads to a possible diagnosis, which points to the type of intervention that is appropriate, and monitoring provides oversight of progress. These are not the sole functions of assessment, but they are of primary importance. Similarly, when an intervention is taking place, ongoing monitoring is part of the progress. Assessment comes from various sources: observations by parents and families, analysis of environmental contexts, specialist observations by professionals, standardized tests and other more criterion referenced measures. Figure 1.1 (p. 3) illustrates how outcomes for a child, accurately assessed with strong intervention, involves a triad of variables.

This figure has been modified since the mid-1980s when Keogh and Sugden (1985) proposed it as a way in which motor development could be described. It was introduced and further developed by Newell (1986) and the Newell model has provided the basis for other research into motor development and impairment (e.g. Hayward and Getchell 2001). We utilize this model.

It is then a short step to take this into assessment and intervention field for children with movement difficulties. The model shows that assessment is not just about the child resources but involves the collection of information from a number of sources and takes account of the ecology of the child in context (Sugden and Henderson 2007). This is then translated into a holistic approach to intervention. This approach is used in the book by Davis and Broadhead (2007), titled *An Ecological Approach to Task Analysis and Movement*.

## The unit of analysis is the child, the task and the environment

All children bring to both the assessment and movement context a set of resources. We portray them as resources rather than deficits as there will almost certainly be strengths as well as weaknesses. Children present with a range of strengths and weaknesses in motor, linguistic, emotional, social, perceptual and cognitive skills and competencies. Children with similar motor skills may differ in other personal characteristics, such as resilience and motivation, and so assessment, support and intervention will reflect these. We use all these resources when developing assessment and intervention protocols. A picture of the child's resources comes from formal assessment procedures and informal observations from therapists, parents and others.

The *environmental context* can include health and educational policy at government and local level, or specific access to services in school, including recreational and health services. The questions are then asked how are the various environmental contexts organized to ensure optimal participation and how does the community make it easy for children with motor difficulties to participate? This is to analogous Bronfenbrenner's (1986) model of an ecological range of influences from macro to micro level. What this means in practice is that the environmental context is a driver to a child's **participation** rate. We know that a crucial part of a child's learning comes from the amount of time on task and that this time on task is hugely influenced by participation, a theme we return to later in this text. We need to understand how access to the environment promotes participation, which can be monitored as part of assessment, and how it is involved in intervention.

The third part of the model involves *task choice and manner of presentation*. Here we are involved in the therapist/teacher/parent–child learning environment and the following questions arise: What are the tasks that will address the child's needs? How are they to be presented in therapy and teaching? How often should 'sessions' take place? What can others, such as parents, do outside of any 'formal' sessions? This is where intervention is inextricably linked to the assessment process. There is a great deal of literature from the general motor learning area about how skills are acquired and we can apply this to children with movement difficulties. One important area here is that of generalization or transfer. Because there is not enough time to teach a child every desirable skill, teaching for transfer becomes a priority. In daily life we are constantly faced with novel situations and true learning is required to address these. Again, the literature on this topic is mainly from the adult motor learning area, but this can be tailored to children with movement difficulties. We describe this in Chapters 2, 6 and 7.

The most important part of the model is that it is dynamic with all parts changing over time in a constantly evolving manner. **The unit of analysis is not the child, nor the task presentation, nor the environmental context, but all three transacting over time**. From this perspective, assessment and intervention are construed in an ecological setting that operates in a self-organizing, often unpredictable fashion, with ever-changing movement dynamics that go beyond its constituent parts.

For us, the terms **assessment** and **intervention** do not quite capture the essence of the whole process. The **collection of information** is a term used by Sugden and Henderson in their text *Ecological Intervention* (2007) and the context, is wider than just assessment. Similarly, the **context for participation rates** and **learning strategies** are broader than simply intervention. However, for custom and practice we will use the terms assessment and intervention noting that we are actually looking at a continuum of activities that starts with collecting information about the child and the context; this information is used to plan a support structure involving multiple individuals and contexts, putting the structure into action and monitoring progress. This information is used to plan a support structure involving multiple individuals and contexts, putting the support structure into action and monitoring progress.

### Purposes of assessment

We have noted that assessment involves collecting information about the child and the environmental context. Burton and Millar (1998), modified by Sugden and Wade (2013), describe the functions of assessment in the following manner (see Box 3.1).

### The benefits of consistent and agreed upon assessment

Consistent and agreed upon assessment helps researchers and clinicians world-wide ensure that they are identifying similar children. This is essential, particularly when in many parts of the world movement disorders are now seen as a primary learning disability. One has only took at the participation rates in the World Developmental Coordination

> **Box 3.1** Purposes of assessment
>
> ✓ Consistent and agreed upon procedures ensuring similar children identified.
> ✓ Diagnosis and categorization of the child leading to services and support.
> ✓ Planning intervention for the child.
> ✓ Assessment that provides an overview of the type of environments the child in which is situated.
> ✓ Enabling feedback to be given to significant others.
> ✓ Assessment is used to evaluate a particular intervention.
> ✓ Examining the child over time to determine what changes have taken place.

Disorder conferences that started in London in the 1990s with around 40 participants from three to four countries, through to the conferences in Toulouse in 2015 and Perth in 2017 that drew together over 200 participants from over 30 countries, to recognize this growth and change. Consistency in diagnosis through accurate assessment gives us better and bigger data to drive our practice.

*Possible diagnosis for support and services*
In many countries, a formal evaluation and diagnosis is required so that health and educational services can be provided. A good example of this is the International Guidelines for Developmental Coordination Disorder (DCD) initiated by Rainer Blank and involving numerous international individuals (Blank et al. 2012, 2019). A label such as DCD allows clinicians to understand the condition and provides a care pathway. It also gives interested parties, such as parents, a sense of community and empowerment, a greater understanding of the disorder and access to support groups with others in a similar situation. The possible effects of low expectancy and exclusion can be eliminated with understanding and good practice. Even if a formal diagnosis is not applied to a child, it does not mean that intervention and support should not take place. Accurate assessment will aid in any support that is given in the home and in schools, outside of any formal procedures.

*Collecting information on the child to plan a learning support programme*
This will involve assessment of the child from numerous sources and an evaluation of the narrower contexts, such as opportunities at school. The information on the child comes from standardized tests, criterion referenced checklist, reports from teachers, parents and others and, wherever possible, from the child. School and home contexts are noted to provide information on opportunities for effective and real participation. These are then combined into an effective care and skill programme.

*Evaluating the environmental context to promote participation*
Here the context of the child is described in more detail with community opportunities, home routines and total educational and health provision and opportunities. We agree

with Bernheimer and Keogh's (1995) assertion that without a partnership between services and home life, the success of intervention will be limited. Participation is crucial to learning as we know that time on task is a major influencing variable affecting final learning outcomes. In order to promote participation, information on the current situation at home, in educational establishments and the community provides the baseline for this work.

*Providing feedback to significant others and the child*
Assessment and intervention results and comments should be fed back to interested parties who, in turn, should be able to give their views to those providing support. It is a community effort with multiple pieces of information fed back in a manner that is comprehensive and easy to follow. This feedback should be given to the child in a manner that is easily understood and can be worked on by the child.

*Evaluating an intervention and support system*
Evaluation can be done at a formal and informal level. Parents can give valuable information regarding both the status of the child (assessment) and how the intervention and support is progressing. In addition, it is essential that the child gives feedback on how successful he or she feels the support and intervention has been. This is combined with the more formal evaluations involving standardized tests. Together they can give a strong overview of the whole assessment–intervention process.

*Analysing changes over time*
Children change both as a result of any support and intervention and through typical development. This change is rarely linear but is dynamic and so frequent measures can monitor the change over time. Change from the various assessment measures can also be placed alongside any change in the environmental context. Monitoring progress over time in regular intervals is recommended by Adolph et al. (2008) who note that infrequent sampling often misses or obscures patterns of development and learning.

These aims and purposes for assessment overlap in part with intervention, thus confirming our view that the support package is one item with several interrelated parts. It is also a dynamic system with a small change in one part creating bigger changes in the total system.

## Bases and types of evidence for intervention

In both educational and health care circles the plea is always for an evidence base for any kind of programme. Whether we are discussing specialist treatments for a heart condition or looking at the best ways to teach numeracy to children, evidence is being sought.

Sugden and Dunford (2007) provided a short guide of what constitutes evidence for working with children with movement difficulties .They proposed that there are three types of evidence, sometimes overlapping but for ease of understanding are presented as three separate areas. Here we simply describe what is involved in each area, they are more fully evaluated in Chapter 6.

*Theory*
The first of these pieces of evidence would fall into what could be called the **theoretical underpinnings**. From what theoretical premise is an intervention approach basing its recommendations? We accept that the word 'theory' can have several interpretations. For example, if one takes an approach such as Sensory Integration Therapy (SIT), its roots and principles can be found in the work done on information processing in the 1960s and taken into the practical field by such practitioners as Jean Ayres (1979). Information processing approaches view individuals as information seekers via senses such as vision and kinaesthesis. This information is transformed through cognitive processes to a motor component leading to the finished action. The primary theoretical base for this approach is the view that perception is indirect and requires translation through a series of operations into action. In addition to SIT, other approaches using similar theoretical idea have emerged, such as kinaesthetic training, which has been developed over the years and has had a widespread influence in occupational therapy (Laszlo and Bairstow 1985).

Another example comes from taking the information-processing model a step further with cognitive decision-making being the focus. An example of this is, Cognitive Orientation to daily Occupational Performance (CO-OP; Polataijko and Mandich 2004). In this approach, cognition is the basis of the intervention process with problem solving on the part of the child being an essential feature. Other, earlier programmes have utilized this concept (Henderson and Sugden 1992; Larkin and Parker 2002).

A third theoretical stance is taken by some researchers who, while not abandoning the cognitive model, place more emphasis on the motor aspect of movement difficulties. This is based on the work by Bernstein (1967) on coordinative structures, degrees of freedom (DoF) in movements and the view of Gibson (1979) that perception is meaningful and direct (not indirect) and involves affordances (opportunities for action). This places more emphasis on the child–context interaction being the unit of analysis and not simply the child. Some researchers are starting to base their work on a more ecological approach with the triad of influences as shown in Figure 1.1 (p. 3). These approaches are reviewed in Chapter 6. The main point here is that any assessment procedure and intervention programme should be underpinned by strong theoretical evidence that provides principles that can be translated into practice.

*Empiricism*

The second pieces of evidence are those obtained through some form of **empirical research**. It is interesting to note that these pieces of evidence are very often the ones that are taken to be the most important. They are used in decision making, in requests for funding and in advising interested parties. The studies vary in type. There are studies using quasi-experimental designs, popular in medicine and psychology, often employing randomized controlled trials (RCT). These RCTs are considered to provide the strongest evidence and many health and educational services base their programmes on their results. Sample groups are selected from a given population and randomly assigned to differing intervention approaches. They are tightly controlled and usually employ skilled professionals to carry out the intervention protocols. Much of our empirical work comes from these types of studies and the results of many of the studies are reviewed in meta-analyses that together often give a stronger indication of the validity of particular types of interventions. Examples of these meta-analyses and/or meta-reviews can be seen in the following papers: Pless and Carlsson 2000; Wilson 2005; Polataijko and Cantin 2006; Blank et al. 2012; Smits-Engelsman et al. 2013; Wilson et al. 2013, 2018; Miyahara et al. 2016; Preston et al. 2016. Other quasi-empirical measures are those where the research is conducted in the field, either in clinics or in schools. The evidence from these is not usually as internally robust as that from RCTs but it has the advantage of having a more ecologically valid setting. Figure 3.1 illustrates the pros and cons of the more experimental types of studies versus more field/experiential oriented studies. When we look at the more experimental data such as RCTs and other methods, we can see that they are internally very robust. Most of the variables are controlled such that bias from

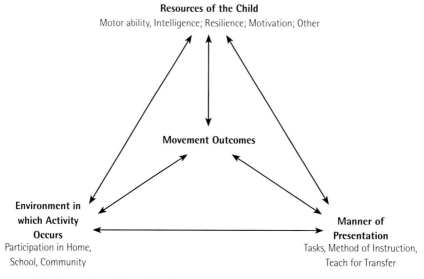

**Figure 3.1** The dynamic relationship between the three factors that influence a movement outcome.

| Box 3.2 Research designs for assessment and intervention | | |
| --- | --- | --- |
| *Types of Studies* | *Advantages* | *Disadvantages* |
| *Quasi experimental* | *Control of internal variables* | *Less ecologically valid* |
| *Continuum* | | |
| *Field studies* | *Strong ecological validity* | *Less control over variables* |

them is kept to a minimum. The drawback of these studies is that they are often more laboratory based and are less ecologically valid with respect to real life situations. The field studies have pros and cons that are the opposite of the experimental ones. They tend to be more ecologically valid, being conducted in the field, such as at home or in school, but with the resultant complication that not all the variables can be adequately controlled. The recent International Consensus Statement (Blank et al. 2019) shows results of empirical studies and provides some guidelines for use in our interventions.

As Box 3.2 shows, this division between the types of studies is not discrete but one that is a continuum moving in dimensions and often with hybrids.

*Professional practice*
A third type of evidence that should be noted is what we have called **professional evidence.** This is evidence we hear from practitioners in the field who are working in support and intervention on a daily basis. They are expert in what they do and have much practical knowledge of the types of support they give. In addition, they are great observers of movement and in informal sessions can note movement activities that cannot be elicited by other means. This type of evidence is strong, and often idiosyncratic to the professional, but is rarely offered in 'official' capacities and, unfortunately, only in discussions at clinic meetings or in staffrooms or workshops. Therefore, we are putting out a plea for more of this type of information to be communicated in a way that will add to the cohort of knowledge that we have. To be included in this are the reports from parents and other close friends and family. They are professional in that they see the child on a daily basis, they can make good comparisons with other children and they have a keen vested interest in the accuracy of their observations. We believe this is very important and, therefore, in Chapter 8 we describe the views and practices of renowned professionals in this field.

Unfortunately, it is not common to have the three types of evidence we have for support and intervention line up in agreement. Our plea is for a more coordinated approach to evaluating research that takes in more than one type of evidence, possibly in the manner we have outlined. In this way we can move confidently and seamlessly from theory through empiricism to practice.

## Biology, cognition constraints and behaviour

A model that has proved useful in looking at developmental disorders in general is one proposed originally by Morton and Frith (1999) and elaborated in 2004 by Morton. Morton's model has been useful in describing and explaining the journey from biology, through cognition, to behaviour in developmental disorders. The model was modified in 2013 by Sugden and Wade to illustrate developmental coordination disorder (see Chapter 1 and Figure 1.1, p. 3).

The model by Morton illustrates how the biological substrates of brain functions and/ or familial genetic characteristics influence cognitive behaviour and, subsequently, child behaviour. Although this model can give us some understanding of behaviour, it is not complete and added feedback loops from the various sections would show how behaviour could influence cognition and ultimately brain mechanisms. Figure 3.2 shows how this would work.

The new model holds that it is not simply cognition that influences motoric behaviour, in this case DCD, but that it involves a number of variables that work in a dynamic and bidirectional manner. Thus, we see in Figure 3.2 (Sugden and Wade 2013) that the three areas of interest interact with each other and the middle variable, instead of being cognitive, involves other variables that are peculiar to movement. These are labelled as constraints by Newell (1986) and will involve such items as coordinative structures, limb DoF, both major bases of coordination.

One can speculate how this model can be used as a basis for both assessment and intervention. In assessment, for example, behaviour has always been central to any description of the difficulties a child has. They are involved in both criteria A and B of the DSM-5 (APA 2013) diagnosis of DCD and would be central to any account of movement difficulties in any other developmental disorder. The DSM-5 notes that these behaviours include delayed motor milestones, problems with cutlery, assembling puzzles, building models, playing ball games, handwriting, with later difficulties in riding a bicycle and driving, all activities of daily living.

**Biology**
Genetics/familial/neuromuscular/birth events

**Constraints**
Organizmic, environmental, task (Newell 1986)
Degrees of freedom, coordinative structures, memory, attention, perception–action

**Behaviour**
Self care skills, recreational skills, fine and gross motor skills, classroom skills

**Figure 3.2** Proposed causal modelling of developmental coordination disorder. Adapted from Morton (2004) by Sugden and Wade (2013).

We already utilize the central part of the modified Morton model by looking at perceptual, attention and certain cognitive skills. What we do not know, as yet, in detail in children with movement difficulties is the area of coordination itself, i.e. how muscles and joints are pulled together to act as a single unit to form smooth skilled movements. This area also has major implications for intervention for how a child is taught or how therapy is given to improve coordination. It has implications as well for how instruction is given, how demonstrations are portrayed, and how the results of a movement are fed back. As we have already noted and will also later elaborate on in Chapter 6, in the first phase of learning a skill, the DoF are often 'frozen' or restricted, enabling the child to achieve some level of control. As the child progresses, the DoF are released, enabling adaptive movements to be incorporated. These change as the child moves through the learning process. Details of these are found in Chapter 6.

The biological aspect of the model is also important for assessment. For example, in DSM-5 criterion D for DCD, DSM-5 criterion D implies DCD has no known neurological problems affecting movement, such as a child with cerebral palsy. There are some debateable issues with regard to the difference between mild cerebral palsy and severe DCD that are often difficult to discern. Yet, in the area of biology we are starting to obtain better information on genetics, on familial issues and more detailed neurological evidence from functional magnetic resonance imaging and other studies (e.g. Zwicker et al. 2009, 2010; Wilson et al. 2017).

The position we are promoting is that a model such as the modified one of Morton's original is a useful template that can guide us when we are making decisions about assessment and intervention. What are we measuring when we assess the child and what are we trying to do when we provide support and intervention? In the case of the latter, are we trying to reorganize the central nervous system? Are we attempting to give the child more problem-solving skills? Are we trying to improve fundamental coordination that will transfer across skills? Are we attempting to simply teach observable behaviours that are skills of everyday living? The same questions can be asked of assessment about what exactly we are evaluating. These questions all point to an answer that involves multiple components acting synergistically to give a more complete picture of the child within her or his environment.

## Validity and reliability

These twin concepts are essential parts of all our practices involving assessment and intervention. Strong validity and reliability give us confidence that our data are robust and trustworthy. A short outline of each is given below. Readers advised to read Burton and Miller (1998) for more detail.

## Validity

The validity of an instrument involves whether the instrument measures what it purports to. If we are trying to measure or improve coordination, how do we know we are addressing the concept? When discussing test construction, and thereby assessment and indeed intervention, we usually talk of four types of validity.

### Face validity

Face validity has a common sense feel to it. Does the instrument look as though it is measuring what it purports to? For example, a hand dynamometer seems to be a good face valid measure of hand-grip strength. When trying to improve an ability such as coordination, what type of activities are needed to achieve this end? How do we measure it? Often face validity involves looking and making a clinical judgement. Face validity is relatively simple, so at times we need something more exact and scientific.

### Construct validity

Any test should have a theoretical background to it to show how the test was constructed. What are the theoretical constructs underlying any test such that they can be distinguished from other constructs? Professional opinion and various forms of factor analysis are often used to confirm whether the test has an appropriate construct.

### Content validity

This type of validity is a check to ensure that the contents of any test cover the full range of the construct described. If one had a test of motor ability that did not include some form of manual skill, one could conclude that the content validity was low.

### Criterion validity

This form of validity has two components: *concurrent* and *predictive*. *Concurrent* validity is a measure compared against a known established standard, such as an already used existing test. *Predictive* validity involves comparing a measure against some later behaviour such as the continuation, or otherwise, of a condition.

## Reliability

Reliability is concerned with how consistent a measure is. If a test is inconsistent it cannot be reliable as there is an uncontrolled variability somewhere that is influencing results. On the other hand, one can have a test that has poor validity but can have high reliability in that the test can be consistently assessing the wrong thing! Reliability is judged by how consistently an instrument can be administered or how internally consistent items in the measure are to each other. It can be traced to three areas: the person taking the test, the test itself and the administration of the test.

*Test-retest reliability*

Test-retest reliability examines how consistently the same person can give the same measure on two or more different occasions. The tester must decide how long the interval should be between the tests. With children, if it is too short, they may remember the items and if it is too long then development that could influence the results may have taken place. Correlation is usually the statistic employed in these cases with a high correlation attesting to the reliability.

*Inter-observer reliability*

Inter-observer reliability measures the concordance between two observers looking at the child at the same time on various measures. Both test-retest and inter-observer measures examine consistency of the tester.

*Internal consistency*

In contrast to the two items above, consistency within the test is examined by looking at how the various items in the test are consistent with each other, i.e. how the measurement reflects one basic dimension. Cronbach's alpha coefficient is often used to estimate consistency in standardized tests (Cronbach 1951).

Many factors contribute to reliability: it could be the performer with age, sex or temporary variables such as fatigue and motivation. It is unwise to conclude that a reliability measure on one age or sex will be the same for another. Test administration is often a concern for assessing reliability, with the test setting and/or experience of the examiner being factors. Burton and Miller (1998) make the point that when assessing balance on a balance beam or standing on one foot; the outcome can be affected by how far the child is from a wall, as when the child gets closer to the wall the effect of optical flow becomes more powerful. This is another example of the context being the unit of analysis and not solely the child. A summary of reliability is shown in Box 3.3.

| **Box 3.3** Reliability and validity | |
|---|---|
| **Validity** | |
| *Face/logical* | *the performance is the measure under question from a common-sense view.* |
| *Construct* | *the relationship of the test to a conceptual framework.* |
| *Content* | *the content covers the variable under question with no extra or missing ones.* |
| *Criterion* | *concurrent-compare to established measure. Predictive-examine against later outcome.* |
| **Reliability** | |
| *Inter-rater* | *agreement between two or more assessors.* |
| *Test-retest* | *agreement of same person at two or more different times.* |
| *Internal consistency* | *measures how well the test items are internally consistent with each other.* |

To obtain a complete picture of a child we would always include the informal observations we have discussed earlier. They may not be as objective as these more formal methods but informal, subjective views from individuals who know the child should always be taken be taken into consideration to complete the picture.

## Participation and learning

These two concepts work together, bidirectionally affecting each other. On the one hand, participation is essential for learning to take place and in motor learning, as in other fields, is a crucial variable for learning. With enhanced, appropriate participation, learning will increase leading the child to gain more resources with which to engage in further participation. This cycle of participation and learning continues.

### *Participation*
Participation is a prerequisite for learning and, as we know from other fields (e.g. reading), time spent on appropriate practice is a hugely influential variable for learning. Time spent on practice, to a large extent, depends upon enabling participation and for children to participate the environment must be accommodating and inviting.

We also know that active participation is important for physical well-being as it is associated with increased self-esteem, self-competence and respect from others. Participation leads to greater happiness and enjoyment of life and is important for developing friendships. Children with movement difficulties participate less than their typically developing peers, thus widening the skill gap. This gap broadens over time, especially in girls. Children with movement difficulties enjoy participation less and parents are less satisfied with outcomes, bringing, in turn, spin-off deficits such as poorer peer relations and lower self-concept and self-worth. These results have been confirmed in several studies such as Mandich et al. 2003; Cairney et al. 2009; and Magalhaes et al. 2011. This trend has been extended by Rosenblum et al. (2017), who found that 4- to 6-year-olds with DCD were poorer than aged-matched peers on activities and participation, interpersonal interactions and executive function control. This indicates that this deficit may start early.

Despite this finding, much can be remedied by altering the participation variables through building activities into daily life, not just in special sessions. Examples would include food preparation and clearing up, gardening, family walks, cycling and other leisure pursuits. Family events and outings involving various types of participation in physical activities may facilitate life-long participation. Schools should be obliged to make reasonable adjustments to their lessons, offering more encouragement and opportunities to all children, with full participation built into the first principles of school policy in all subjects, particularly science and technology and physical education. In health services, the questions surround how to use professional expertise to support teachers and empower parents. One method could be by using different practices and scheduling to best fit the client's needs, such as incorporating group work for example. The community can also become involved with sports centres encouraged to actively seek children with difficulties, rather than having a caring, yet passive, welcoming policy.

By modifying the environment in different ways, we accumulate small yet significant increases in participation and by increasing enjoyable participation we have a child on task for more time, actively involved in more appropriate practice. We can then look to making small changes in the learning process from many different angles. Chen and Cohen (2003) describe how participation is a function of school variables (policies and training), community opportunities (leisure activity choices and attitudes) and home context (family life, culture and daily routines).

It is interesting to note that the resources of the child, or their deficits, are not the only variables that affect how much a child can participate. Participation is a variable that can be influenced by macro and micro societal alterations. The answer lies in the hands of the professionals, not the child.

*Learning*

One common definition of learning is that it is **a set of internal processes leading to a relatively permanent change in the capability for skilled behaviour associated with practice and experience** (Schmidt and Lee 1999, p. 264). In Chapter 2 we outlined what the progression of learning involves and the practice variables that affect it.

If we deconstruct this concept, we first note that learning is a set of internal processes that infer that you cannot *see* learning, only the results of learning through observed performance. Capturing numerous performances at different times might be indicative of learning. In addition, a relatively permanent change implies that learning is not a temporary phenomenon; and while performance may drop a little, the permanent capability remains and can, with practice, restore the performance more quickly than when it was initially learned. It is associated with **practice and experience,** with practice being formal, such as an occupational therapy session, and experience involving less formality, drawing upon everyday activities.

*Learning outcomes*

As we noted in Chapter 2, and above, learning is measured by observing multiple performances over time. In handwriting, for example, it can involve any or a combination of the following:

- *Improvement/accomplishment in performance*
  A child can now perform a skill or perform it better than previously. A child with slow handwriting improves in speed and legibility to such as extent that such activities as taking notes for homework are no longer a problem.

- *Consistency and stability in performance*
  The handwriting can be done quickly, whether copying from text, whiteboard, or listening to someone and taking notes. A more adaptable, quicker performance results, even when having to view different forms of writing.

- *Component tasks become whole*
  The child integrates all the actions in handwriting, so they become one rather than a set of component parts. The unit moves from letter, to word, to phrase, and so on.

- *Performance becomes more automatic.*
  The child no longer has to think about the parts of handwriting but can write at the same time as thinking about the content and the next sentence.

- *Flexible use of freezing and freeing degrees of freedom*
  The child can write in various positions: sitting at a desk, writing on a whiteboard, writing on the school bus, all demanding different sets of coordinative structures or muscle and joint configurations in order to complete the task.

These are examples of how we can measure performance in a more fine-grained manner. Through these and other examples we can better measure the progress that has been made and set goals for support and intervention.

*Learning progressions*

Daily learning progresses in an individual in various phases: accelerations, plateaus and sharp steps in between, as shown by the examples of learning curves in Figure 2.1 and as described in Chapter 2. These progressions have been studied extensively in many other fields of activity.

Four are shown again here but there are many more. Figure 2.1a shows linear progression, which tends to be rare. Figure 2.1b shows learning to be negatively accelerated with fast learning at the start followed by a slowing later. This is usual of a typical person learning a moderately difficult task. It is consistent over a range of tasks, both fine and gross motor. Figure 2.1c shows learning to be positively accelerated with slow learning at first followed by an acceleration later when the individual has 'got the hang of' the task.

This type of curve is often seen with those who have some form of difficulty or with a difficult task. Figure 2.1d shows a changing acceleration, with a slow start followed very fast progress eventually slowing down. It is useful to remember that these learning curves are really performance curves representing performance at various times during the practice process.

These learning progressions or stages have been divided into parts for ease of explanation, but it is important to remember that they are not discrete stages but continuous along various dimensions. A number of models of learning progressions have been proposed and are described in Chapter 2. An early example, and one that is probably used as much as any other, is the one proposed by Fitts and Posner in 1967. In this model the progressions are divided into three stages: cognitive, associative and autonomous. Here, the performer starts by getting to know what the task demands followed by a trial and error stage with feedback showing gradual improvement. The third stage becomes automatic with the performer not having to think about the task too much but can perform another task at the same time or plan for a more complex solution to a movement problem.

Other researchers have slightly different, but complementary, views on progression. Gentile (2000) has proposed a **two-stage model.** This first stage appears to be a combination of Fitts' and Posner's first two stages, in getting to know the task and environmental demands, resulting in improvement over trials. In Gentile's second stage the performer becomes more consistent, more adaptable and uses less effort in more complex situations.

A third model is the **dynamic systems view of learning** described by Bernstein (1967) and Gibson (1979), which has been elaborated on by the work of (Kelso (1979); Turvey (1990). Here the emphasis is on controlling the coordination dynamics from freezing to freeing DoF. To achieve this, muscles and joints are gradually combined into coordinative structures that are softly assembled and attune to the environmental context. In the early stages of learning, the individual uses as few DoF as possible (i.e. they freeze them). As learning progresses the individual frees the DoF allowing increased flexibility to meet the demands of a changing environments. Therapists use this concept in their work, asking individuals to fix some body parts (freeze the DoF) and then show ways to release them to meet environmental demands (freeing the DoF). This is a complex area and more recent work has shown that it is better to keep some DoF constant, such as in violin playing (Konzack et al. 2009). This is another example of the child in context with the task being the unit of analysis rather than simply the child.

All three explanations have common elements, the main one being that learning progresses sometimes evenly and at other times in fits and starts, all depending on the task,

---

**Box 3.4** The learning progression

**Fitts and Posner:**

✓ **Cognitive stage** – understanding the requirements of the task

✓ **Associative stage** – practice, trial and error and feedback

✓ **Autonomous stage** – almost automatic leading to multi-tasking

**Gentile:**

✓ **Stage 1** – Learning appropriate coordination pattern to context demand. Discriminate essential from non-essential parts of the environment.

✓ **Stage 2** – Aims for adaptability and consistency of effort and distinguishes between closed and open skills.

**Dynamic Systems:** Bernstein (1967), Turvey et al. (1978), Whiting (1984), Newell (1986) Thelen (1995)

✓ **Freezing degrees of freedom** – to enable some accomplishment of task

✓ **Freeing degrees of freedom** – to enable adaptability to more complex environmental demands

✓ **Enhancing perception** – action linkages

---

the environmental context and the resources of the learner as we show in Figure 1.1 (p. 3). A summary of the different accounts of learning progression is shown in Box 3.4.

## Conclusion

This chapter lays the foundation for the more practical guidelines outlined in Chapters 4 to 7 and is linked to Chapter 2 that provided the theoretical and empirical evidence from the motor learning literature. Here we have outlined how we see assessment and intervention, namely (1) collecting information to cover assessment; (2) participation that enables maximum time on task and satisfaction; and (3) learning via successive performances, which shows progression over time.

However, it is highly appropriate that we modify and scale our instructions, demonstrations, explanations and feedback to fit the learning stage achieved by the child. In this regard, we need to ask the following questions: how do we present the learning context to the child as they progress through the learning process? What do we say to the child when the first task is introduced? How do we coordinate our instructions with any demonstrations we may show; how do we provide initial feedback in the first instance? As the child progresses through the various learning phases how do instructions, demonstrations, and feedback change to account for this progression? These issues will be discussed in the next four chapters.

# References

Adolph KE, Robinson SR, Young JW, Gill Alvarez F (2008) What is the shape of developmental change? *Psychol Rev* 115: 527–543.

APA (2013) *Diagnostic and Statistical Manual of Mental Disorder,* 5th edition (DSM-5) Washington, DC: American Psychiatric Association.

Ayes JR (1979) *Sensory Integration and the Child.* Los Angeles: Western Psychological Services.

Bernheimer LP, Keogh BK (1995) Weaving intervention into the fabric of everyday life: an approach to family assessment. *Topics Early Child Spec Educ* 15: 415–433.

Bernstein N (1967) *The Coordination and Regulation of Movements.* New York: Pergamon Press.

Blank R, Barnett A, Cairney J, et al. (2017) European Academy of Childhood Disability International Clinical Practice Guideline on the definition, diagnosis, assessment, intervention and psycho-social aspects of developmental coordination disorder (DCD), *Long version. Dev Med Child Neurol.*

Blank R, Barnett AL, Cairney J, et al. (2019) International clinical practice recommendations on the definition, diagnosis, assessment, intervention, and psychosocial aspects of developmental coordination disorder. *Dev Med Child Neurol* 61: 242–285.

Blank R, Smits-Engelsman B, Polatajko H, Wilson P (2012) European Academy for Childhood Disability (EACD): recommendations on the definition, diagnosis and intervention of developmental coordination disorder (long version). *Dev Med Child Neurol* 54: 54–93.

Bronfenbrenner U (1986) *The Ecology of Human Development.* Cambridge, MA: Harvard University Press.

Burton AW, Miller DE. (1998) *Movement Skill Assessment.* Champaign IL: Human Kinetics.

Cairney J, Hay JA, Veldhizen S, Missiuna C, Faught BE (2009) Developmental coordination disorder, sex and activity deficit over time: a longitudinal analysis of participation trajectories in children with and without developmental coordination disorder. *Dev Med Child Neurol* 52: 67–72.

Chen HF, Cohn ES (2003) Social participation for children with developmental coordination disorder: conceptual, evaluation and intervention considerations. *Phys Occup Ther Pediatr* 13: 61–78.

Cronbach LJ (1951) Coefficient alpha and the internal structure of tests. *Psychometrika* 16: 297–334.

Davis WE, Broadhead GD (2007) *Ecological Task Analysis and Movement.* Champaign, IL: Human Kinetics.

Fitts PM, Posner M (1967) *Human Performance.* Belmont, CA: Brooks/Cole.

Gentile A (2000) Skill acquisition: action movement and neuro-motor processes. In: Carr J, Shepherd RB (eds). *Movement Science: Foundations for Physical Therapy in Rehabilitation,* 2nd edition. Gaithersberg, MD: Aspen.

Gibson JJ (1979) *The Ecological Approach to Visual Perception.* Boston, MA: Houghton Mifflin.

Hayward KM, Getchell N (2001) *Lifespan Motor Development.* Champaign, IL: Human Kinetics.

Henderson SE, Sugden DA, Barnett AE (2007) *Movement Assessment Battery for Children,* 2nd edition. London: Pearson.

Henderson SE, Sugden DA (1992) *Movement Assessment Battery for Children.* London: Pearson.

Kelso J, Southard D, Goodman D (1979) On the nature of interlimb coordination. *Science* 203: 1029–1031.

Keogh JF, Sugden DA (1985) *Movement Skill Development*. New York: MacMillan.

Konzack J, Vander Veldon J, Jaeger H (2009) Learning to play the violin; motor control by freezing not freeing degrees of freedom. *J Motor Behav* 41: 243–252.

Larkin D, Parker H (2002) 'Task-specific intervention for children with developmental coordination disorder: A systems view. In: Cermack S, Larkin D (eds). *Developmental Coordination Disorder*. Albany NY: Delmar, pp. 234–247.

Laszlo JI, Bairstow P (1985) *The Test of Kinaesthetic Sensitivity*. London: Senkit PTY in association with Holt, Rinehart & Winston.

Mandich AD, Polatajko HJ, Rodger S (2003) Rites of passage: understanding participation of children with developmental coordination disorder. *Hum Mov Sci* 22: 583–595.

Magalhães LC, Cardoso AA, Missiuna C (2011) Activities and participation in children with developmental coordination disorder: a systematic review. *Res Dev Disabil* 32: 1309–1316.

Miyahara M (1994) Subtypes of students with learning disabilities based upon gross motor functions. *Adapt Physl Activ Q* 11: 368–383.

Miyahara M, Lagisz M, Nakagawa S, Henderson SE (2016) A narrative meta-review of a series of systematic and meta-analysis reviews on intervention outcomes for children with developmental coordination disorder. *Child Care Health Dev* 43: 733–742.

Morton J (2004) *Understanding Developmental Disorders*. Oxford: Blackwell.

Morton J, Frith U (1999) Causal modeling: a structural approach to developmental psychopathology. In: Cicchetti D, Cohen DJ (eds). *Developmental Psychopathology, Volume 1: Theory and Methods*. New York: Wiley, pp. 357–399.

Newell KM (1986) Development of coordination. In: Wade MG, Whiting HTA (eds). *Motor Development in Children: Aspects of Coordination and Control. NATO ASI Series D, Behavioural and Social Sciences*. Dordrecht: Martinus Nijhoff, pp. 341–360.

Pless M, Carlsson M (2000) Effects of motor skill intervention on developmental coordination disorder: a meta-analysis. *Adapt Phys Activ Q* 17: 381–401.

Polatajko HJ, Mandich AD (2004) *Enabling Occupation in Children: The Cognitive Orientation to Daily Occupational Performance (CO-OP) Approach*. Ottowa, ON: Canadian Association of Occupational Therapists.

Polatajko H, Cantin N (2006) Developmental coordination disorder (dyspraxia): an overview of the state of the art. *Sem Pediatr Neurol* 12: 250–258.

Preston N, Magallon S, Hill LBJ, Andrews E, Ahern SA, Mon-Williams M (2016) A systematic review of high quality randomized controlled trials investigating motor skill programmes for children with developmental coordination disorder. *Clin Rehab* 31: 857–870.

Rosenblum S, Waissman P, Diamond GW (2017) Identifying play characteristics of pre-school children with developmental ccoordination disorder via parental questionnaires. *Hum Mov Sci* 53: 5–15.

Schmidt RA, Lee TD (1999) *Motor Control and Learning: a Behavioral Emphasis*. Human Kinetics: Champaign IL, p. 264.

Smits-Engelsman BCM, Blank R, Van der Kaay A-C, Mosterd-Van der Meijs R, Polataijko HJ, Wilson PH (2013) Efficacy of interventions to improve motor performance in children with developmental coordination disorder: a combined systematic review and meta-analysis. *Dev Med Child Neurol* 55: 229–237.

Sugden DA, Dunford CD (2007) The role of theory, empiricism and experience in intervention for children with movement difficulties. *Disabil Rehabil* 29: 3–11.

Sugden DA, Henderson SE (2007) *Ecological Intervention.* London: Pearson.

Sugden DA, Wade MG (2013) *Typical and Atypical Motor Development.* Clinics in Developmental Medicine. London: Mac Keith Press.

Thelen (1995) Motor development: a new synthesis. *Am Psychol* 50: 79–95.

Turvey M (1990) Coordination. *American Psychologist*, 45: 938–953.

Turvey MT, Shaw RE, Mace W (1978) Issues in the theory of action: degrees of freedom, coordinative structures and coalitions. In: Requin J (ed.). *Perceiving, Acting and Knowing.* Hillsdale, NJ: Erlbaum, pp. 211–265.

Whiting HTA (1984) *Human Motor Actions: Bernstein Reassessed.* Amsterdam: N. Holland.

Wilson P (2005) Practitioner review: approaches to assessment and treatment of children with DCD: an evaluative review. *J Child Psychol Psychiatry* 46: 806–823.

Wilson PH, Ruddock S, Smits-Engelsman B, Polatajko H, Blank R (2013) Understanding performance deficits in developmental coordination disorder: a meta-analysis of recent research *Dev Med Child Neurol* 55: 217–228.

Wilson PH, Smits Engelsman B, Caeyenberghs K, et al. (2017) Cognitive and neuroimaging findings in developmental coordination disorder; new insights from a systematic review of recent research. *Dev Med Child Neurol* 59: 1117–1129.

Zwicker JG, Missiuna C, Boyd LA (2009) Neural correlates of developmental coordination disorder. *J Child Neurol* 24: 1273–1281.

Zicker JG, Missiuna C, Harris SR, Boyd LA (2010) Brain activation of children with developmental coordination disorder is different than peers. *Pediatrics* 126: 678–686.

# Chapter 4

## Assessment and other information: Case studies

In this chapter, detail is presented on how we move from the general account of assessment described in Chapter 3 to how, in practical situations, information is collected. This information includes various indices of the resources of the child, such as standardized tests and criterion referenced tests, together with qualitative accounts from teachers, parents, other interested parties and the children themselves. The context of the child is included as a variable here as it will later affect the profiles and goals and objectives leading to intervention programmes. Case studies of children with developmental coordination disorder (DCD) are presented here together with additional examples from children with a movement difficulty as a secondary problem, such as in autistic spectrum disorder (ASD) and attention-deficit–hyperactivity disorder (ADHD).

A child may have movement difficulties and yet may not have a formal diagnosis. A formal diagnosis brings with it many advantages, such as recognition that the child *does* have a disorder, which can help parents, professionals and the child. It also enables the child and parents to access resources from education, health services or other agencies. However, while children may have the same diagnostic label, a full description of symptoms, strengths and difficulties is usually more accurate than a diagnostic category alone. Thus, even without a diagnostic label, if a child has a movement difficulty, we believe there is an ethical responsibility to support the child.

### Triad of influences

Assessment of movement difficulties involve a triad of variables that influence movement and other outcomes for the child, whether their development is typical or atypical. It is the metrics within these variables that differ. Thus, an 8-year-old child of with a diagnosis of DCD will fit into this triad in the same way as a young adult with a diagnosis of ASD and movement difficulties. A child with no diagnosis also fits perfectly into the triad. The content of each part of the triad may change, but the triad remains the same. The triad is a dynamic, constantly evolving system with each part influencing the other over time, in a dynamic transaction. Our working figure for the triad is shown in Figure 1.1 (p. 3).

The figure shows that assessment, or more accurately, collecting information, would include gathering information on the resources of the child and the environmental context. These will influence the choice of task and manner of presentation of the intervention.

Individuals working with the child must have a clear idea of what information is needed in order to plan an effective programme of intervention. The programme comes from a variety of information sources that are pulled together into a profile, leading to a set of objectives and an appropriate intervention and support regimen. The information collected will create a picture of the daily life of the child and his or her ecological context so that an appropriate support system can be built into the daily activities of the child. Sugden and Henderson (2007) have called this approach 'Ecological Intervention'. It is an approach that is not simply a set of activities for the child to perform but involves minor restructuring of the child's daily routines, overseen by individuals playing different roles in the child's life.

## Responsible person

In this chapter, we are describing the various ways in which information can be collected about a child, their personal resources and the environmental context in order to choose the types of tasks and presentation that are most appropriate. Naturally, this will involve different types information from multiple sources of. Parents often have reports from various professionals, but they have never been pulled together in a cohesive manner. For this to we recommend that a named person be appointed to coordinate the information. It could be a *Key worker, Movement coach or Navigator*.

In their work on ecological intervention, Sugden and Henderson outline the role of what they call the 'movement coach' to ensure that 'the right things are happening in the right places at the right moment in time … [and the named person] is the person who the child or his or her family see as the main point of contact' (Sugden and Henderson 2007, p. 6). This person would have the responsibilities listed in Box 4.1.

### Candidates for the role
The named person will work with the child, the family members, school personnel, health professionals and community agents. As with all teams, there must be agreement on the common goals and the manner in which these goals are achieved.

---

**Box 4.1** Responsibilities of the movement coach

- ✓ Taking overall responsibility for the child and his/her support needs.
- ✓ Advocating for child's needs and appropriate resources.
- ✓ Liaising with appropriate interested parties: parents, teachers, health professionals and community organizations.
- ✓ Interpreting information from different sources and pulling it together to ensure that it is meaningful for interested parties.
- ✓ Negotiating with parents and professionals to ensure the correct balance for the child and she or he is not overloaded.
- ✓ Sensitivity to the family situation and acting accordingly.
- ✓ Bringing together the various sources of information on the child and the context and facilitating the collation of this information into a meaningful support and intervention plan.

---

As this person is crucial to the whole process of assessment, support and intervention, who should it be?

This is not an easy question to answer, especially with diminishing resources in both health and educational services to fund such a role. The role must be part of their job description, which means that they may need to give up other parts of their job. The role will require adequate resources, but we feel it is a crucial role if the child is to receive the appropriate support in a manner that is acceptable and achievable within their daily life.

Possible candidates for this role include the following:

- A **teacher** in the child's school who has responsibility for special educational needs. The advantages of using a special needs teacher for the role are is that they see the child on a daily basis, are knowledgeable, are aware of the child's needs and have contact with parents. The disadvantage is that the child may be just one of several such children in their portfolio requiring support and that the workload may become overwhelming. Other support teachers may be able help by alleviating this workload but, clearly, a teacher in this role would need additional resources.

- A **health professional**, such as an occupational therapist or physiotherapist, would be appropriate. The advantage of using a therapist would be that they have a specialist knowledge in motor impairment. Disadvantages include the need for additional resources as noted above, and the fact they see the child only occasionally.

- The **parent** has the obvious advantages of seeing the child constantly and knowing him or her well. An added advantage would be that a parent could become a skilled operator in this area and be enabled to pass on their skills to help others. However, a disadvantage would be the subjectivity the parent brings. We believe the parent should be actively involved at all stages of any support process, but care should be taken to involve all others in the process.

We believe that through the efficient and effective use of a named person the child will receive more appropriate support and intervention and, in the long run, have better outcomes. This in turn will bring benefits such as fewer problems later on and a better long-term prognosis, thereby justifying the additional expense of the support process.

The named person will liaise with a team dedicated to supporting the child and will include one or more family members, an education professional such as class teacher or learning support assistant, a health professional, such as an occupational therapist or physical therapist, and a club leader or a local disability officer from the community. The named person will work with these individuals to ensure that each knows the overall goal, their particular role, what to do at any point and who to contact if they have questions. In the following sections we detail how to collect information on the child followed by a description of the available options in the school, health services and community.

### The resources of the child

Each child will present a unique set of resources, even if he or she is described as being in the same diagnostic category as another. The first step, therefore, is to look at who first made the observation that the child was having difficulty with movement. This could be a parent, a teacher, a health professional, particularly in the early years, or the child him or herself. The order in which the various pieces of information are collected will depend to some extent on earlier reports and who has reported the concern. Here we list the information in a logical sequence, but this sequence could change depending on the events leading up to the decision to intervene. Variations in this sequence will be shown in the case studies presented later in the chapter. We emphasize that although children are given diagnostic labels for a variety of reasons, we are concentrating on their strengths and needs that will eventually lead to a profile illustrating the most appropriate support.

### Standardized tests

It is not the aim of this section to weigh up the pros and cons of each standardized test. It is rather to briefly describe the tests that are used most frequently and recommended by independent reviewers and to list others that are used occasionally. The most comprehensive review we have on assessment for children with DCD is the International Consensus Statement by a group of professionals gathered from around the word (Blank et al. 2017). It is expected that this document will be adopted by professionals worldwide. The document involves recommendations for children with DCD and should be viewed in the light of *Diagnostic and Statistical Manual of Mental Disorders,* 5th edition criteria for DCD (DSM-5; APA 2013). The DSM-5 notes that the first criterion for a diagnosis of DCD is that the learning and performance of coordinated motor skills is substantially below that expected of an individual, given their age and opportunities for learning (Criterion A). This is shown by awkwardness and clumsiness in the performance of every day motor skills (APA 2013, p. 74). This criterion is usually assessed by an individual standardized test.

The International Consensus Statement (Blank et al. 2019) notes that the most widely recommended individual tests are the Movement Assessment Battery for Children (MABC-2) (Henderson et al. 2007) and the Bruininks–Oseretsky Test (BOT-2) (Bruininks and Bruininks 2007). Both have strong reliability and validity measures and are used widely by clinicians and researchers. If children with suspected DCD are being assessed, both the above tests would be appropriate for Criterion A.

### The MABC-2

The MABC-2 (Henderson et al. 2007) is a test comprising three sections: a Standardized Test, a Checklist and an Intervention Manual. In this section we present a description of the test. The test (for 3- to 16-year-olds) has three parts – Manual Dexterity, Ball Skills and Balance – and is made up of eight items overall. There are qualitative observations that the clinician can note when the individual is performing the test. Scores and centile ranks can be obtained for the total test, each section, or for individual items. The authors recommend that a score in the lowest 5% indicates that the individual has a current movement difficulty that needs attention. A score from the 5th to the 15th centile indicates that the individual should be monitored closely. The test is used internationally, in both clinical and research settings and standardizations have been made in 15 countries and translated into the corresponding languages.

Details on the reliability and validity of the MABC-2 Test can be found in the Manual and in journal articles. For example, Schultz et al. (2011) performed confirmatory factor analysis on the data from the first edition of the MABC-2 (Henderson et al. 2007). Data from 1172 children across three age bands were used and the findings were that in the younger age group (3–6 years) a complex factor emerged with a general overall factor, as well as specific factors for the three components of the test. This general factor disappeared with age, with only modest correlations between each factor. The authors interpreted this data as confirmation that abilities change both within and between children as they develop.

### The Bruininks–Oseretsky Test

Again, the Bruininks–Oseretsky Test (BOT-2) (Bruininks and Bruininks 2007) is a comprehensive package and contains both a full test and a short-form test; we describe the former here. The BOT-2 consists of items on fine motor precision, fine motor integration, manual dexterity, bilateral coordination, balance, running speed and agility, upper-limb coordination and strength. The test is suitable for individuals aged from 4 to 21 years and has scores and centile ranks for all the test items. The BOT-2 is used worldwide and extensively by clinicians in the USA. Details on the reliability and validity of the BOT-2 can be found in the manual and in journal articles.

Both the MABC-2 and the BOT-2 are recommended for individual assessment with the proviso that they can only be administered by suitably qualified individuals, such as occupational and physiotherapist, educational psychologists and others suitable trained. They both have the endorsement of the International Consensus Statement on DCD (2017).

There are other tests that examine more specific aspects of motor performance. For example, the Detailed Assessment of Speed in Handwriting (DASH) (Barnett et al. 2007, 2009, 2011) includes five subtests, each testing a different aspect of handwriting speed and legibility. The subtests examine fine motor and precision skills, the speed of producing well-known symbolic material, the ability to alter speed of performance on two tasks with identical content and free writing competency.

The DASH assessment identifies words written per minute in relation to national averages, under test and non-test conditions. This gives a more accurate description of why the child is struggling to write legibly and at a normal speed. Standardized subtest and composite scores are provided based on a nationally stratified normative sample of over 500 children collected across the UK in 2006. The DASH is widely used by occupational therapists.

Regarding gross motor skills, there is the popular Test of Gross Motor Development (TGMD-2) (Ulrich 2000). Both DASH and TGMD are useful when examining a particular aspect of a child's performance in more detail.

### Criterion referenced assessments/checklists

These instruments are usually more readily available than the tests described above and can be administered by teachers and often parents, usually in the form of a checklist. They are criterion referenced in that they usually assess whether a child can perform a particular task that often has relevance to activities of daily living. Again, DSM-5 diagnostic criteria for DCD provide some guidance here. Criterion B of the DSM-5 diagnosis notes that the poor motor skills, as noted in Criterion A, have a significant interfering effect on activities of daily living at home, school, leisure and at work. The two checklists that have often been employed in this regard, and which do not have the same restrictive administrative requirements of the standardized tests, are the MABC-2 Checklist (Henderson et al. 2007) and the Developmental Coordination Disorder Questionnaire (DCDQ) (Wilson et al. 2007; Schoemaker and Wilson 2015).

### The MABC Checklist

The MABC Checklist is part of the overall MABC-2 (Henderson et al. 2007) and contains three sections. Section A involves those activities that are performed when the environment is stable and predictable in both space and time. It has 15 items to score divided into three sections of self-care skills, such as fastening buttons; classroom skills, such as using scissors to cut paper; and physical education/recreational skills, such as hopping on either foot. Section B involves those activities where the situation is dynamic or unpredictable. It also has 15 items divided in to three sections of self-care/classroom skills, such as carrying a drink around a busy classroom avoiding moving persons; ball skills, such as continually bouncing and keeping control of a large playground ball; and physical education/recreational skills, such as participating in dodging and chasing games. Section C includes the non-motor factors that might affect movement performance, such as being disorganized, lack of planning and distractibility. The MABC-2 has a scoring system of 1–4 indicating whether the child can perform the given task and is suitable for children between the ages of 5 and 12 years. It uses a 'traffic light' system, with green indicating no current motor problems, amber indicating that the child is between the 5th and 15th centile and has some risk of motor difficulties and a red section, below the 5th centile, indicating the presence of a motor difficulty. Its reliability and validity have been shown to be of the required standard and it has been recommended for use by teachers for screening children with movement difficulties (Schoemaker et al. 2003, 2012).

### The Developmental Coordination Disorder Questionnaire

The Developmental Coordination Disorder Questionnaire (DCDQ) has two versions: the first for children aged between 5 and 15 years and the second (Little DCDQ) for children aged between 3 and 5 years. Both were developed in Canada at the Alberta Children's Hospital (Wilson et al. 2007; Schoemaker and Wilson 2015), and both are aimed primarily at parents of children with movement difficulties. The original DCDQ has 15 items divided into three sections: control during movement, such as throwing a ball and running; fine motor/handwriting, such as writing fast and cutting; and general coordination, such as learning new skills. Each item is scored on a scale of 1–5 as to whether a particular description fits the child. The scoring system divides children into the two groups: 'probably not DCD' and 'suspected DCD'.

The International Consensus Statement (Blank et al. 2019) notes that the DCDQ is the best supported of the questionnaires, with psychometric property studies underway (Wilson et al. 2014). The questionnaire was studied with the parents of 287 typically developing children. Logistic regression modelling was used to generate separate cut-off scores for three age groups (overall sensitivity, 85%; overall specificity, 71%). The DCDQ was then compared to other standardized measures in a sample of 232 clinically-referred children. Differences in scores on the DCDQ between children with and without coordination problems provide evidence of construct validity. Concurrent validity was evident with the MABC-2 and with the Visual Motor Integration (VMI). It also has the important advantage of being reasonably short and easy to complete by parents and others.

The Little Developmental Coordination Questionnaire (LDCDQ) (Wilson et al. 2014; Schoemaker and Wilson 2015) is a parent report measure that screens for motor coordination difficulties in 3- and 4-year-old children. It consists of 15 items that are grouped into gross motor skills and fine motor skills.

The gross motor section contains items such as throwing, catching and running, while the fine motor skills include threading, cutlery usage and placing stickers. The LDCDQ measures functional skills in several contextual areas across home and preschool environments and during play activities. It has good test–retest reliability and internal consistency. Construct validity was supported by a factor analysis and a significant difference in scores of children who were typically developing but at risk of developing DCD. Concurrent validity was also high. Discriminant function analysis showed that all 15 items were able to distinguish the two groups. The LDCDQ correlates well with the MABC-2 and VMI.

Both the DCDQ and MABC-2 have satisfactory reliability and validity and can be used by parents, teachers or anyone who is in close contact with the child. Neither should be used to formally diagnose a condition such as DCD, but both provide useful information on the child's overall profile.

Other checklists that are used include the Early Years Movement Checklist (Chambers and Sugden 2002, 2006) for children aged 3–5 years. This comprises four sections: self-help, desk skills, general classroom skills and recreational/playground skills. It can be used by parents, carers and teachers. For adults, much of the work has been done by Kirby et al. (2008) on their Adult Checklist. A full report on the assessment instruments can be found in the International Consensus Statement (Blank 2017).

## Parent, teacher, child reports and history taking

Movement difficulties come in a variety of forms and are contextual. For that reason other assessment methods need to be considered that will add to the overall of information on the child's resources.

### Parental reports

First, we strongly believe in the value of parental reports. Parents have the advantage of seeing the child every day in a variety of movement situations. Their continual observations should be considered whenever information is being collected on a child. Without the cooperation of the parents in any support situation, the chances of success are limited (Bernheimer and Keogh 1995). These informal, continuing observations of the child in

> **Box 4.2** Reasons for referral and presenting problems
>
> ✓ Family history – to include the presence of developmental disorders or other genetic conditions.
> ✓ Medical history – to include information about major accidents, diseases, neurological disorders, psychological disorders and sensory problems.
> ✓ Developmental and educational history – to include information about pregnancy, birth, milestones, achievements, social contacts, kindergarten, school, grade levels, history of motor engagement, family habits, home environment and access to motor activities.
> ✓ Impact of the condition – including that on activities of daily living.
> ✓ Contextual factors such as the amount and type of previous intervention and support; description of current family structure; friendship groups and relationship status (social support, living with partner, etc.) and socio-economic status.
> ✓ Ongoing observations that the parent makes on the child in the course of daily living.

the course of daily life are an essential feature from which an ecological approach can be developed. Possible contents of a parent report are shown in Box 4.2.

*School reports*
Teachers typically see the child on a daily basis, particularly in primary schools, in several different situations, and have the advantage of having other children in the classroom as comparisons.

Parents and teachers can provide valuable qualitative information on the child that can be fed into his or her overall profile and used to construct an intervention and support programme. Both sources of information provide detail on the child's strengths and areas of need that will produce a more accurate profile leading to appropriate intervention and support. In some situations we have noticed the separation of school reports from those of health services. We would make a plea for these to be combined so that the care and support package is based on information from all available sources.

*Child reports*
An important source of information is the child. The more input the child has into what happens to him or her the more likely he or she is to be cooperative and put effort into the process and outcomes. The way information can be obtained from the child varies with the individual. The older and more verbal the individual the more he or she can articulate their concerns and what they would like to see in any support system. Even with younger children this can be done by careful questioning and by using cards and pictures that illustrate various situations. This is taken further when we examine the objectives an individual prefers. A system such as Perceived Efficacy

and Goal Setting System (PEGS) (Missiuna et al. 2004), is a good example of a model that allows a child (in this case 6–9y) to identify those tasks in which there is a difficulty and set goals needed for support. The child is asked what they see as a difficulty, if any, and what kind of priority they place on the various activities they are asked to perform in everyday living.

*History taking*
The International Consensus Statement on DCD (2017) confirms the above recommendations and recommends careful history taking which should include the following:

- Evaluation documents: recent reports of others (nursery, school, therapist, other family members); reports concerning motor functions, activities/participation, environmental factors, support systems, individual personal factors [International Classification of Functioning, Disability and Health (ICF) framework].

- Reports concerning behaviour that bear on comorbidity for attentional disorders, ASD, learning and language disorders.

- Reports concerning executive function (e.g. strategic planning).

- Reports concerning academic achievement.

- Views of the individual from adapted questionnaires but not fully recommended.

With adolescents and adults, self-reporting would include the following:

- Reasons for referral and presenting problems.

- Family history – developmental disorders.

- Medical history – accidents, diseases, neurological disorders, sensory problems, new symptoms arising, psychological problems and any medication.

- Educational and employment history, schooling, training, work placements and employment; levels of attainment.

- Impact of the condition on daily life.

- Contextual factors – amount and type of any intervention and support, current family structure, relationship status, socio-economic status, and personal resources.

With all children who have a movement difficulty, and where there is a need for a defining diagnosis, we must decide what it is *not* in order to make a definitive statement as to what it is. For example, if we are assessing a child for potential DCD there are both inclusionary criteria (DSM-5 criteria A and B mentioned above) and exclusionary criteria (Criterion D). The exclusionary criteria are in Criterion D in DSM-5 which states that

| Box 4.3 Summary for assessment of child's resources | |
|---|---|
| Standardized tests | Suitably qualified individual |
| Observation | Suitably qualified individual |
| Criterion referenced tests/checklists | Parent, teacher, other |
| Interview reports | Parent, teacher, other |
| Child/adult voice | Child/adult interview |

the problems with motor skills are not better explained by another identifiable neuro-logical condition, such as cerebral palsy (CP) or muscular dystrophy, for example, and are not better explained by an intellectual disability or a visual problem (APA, 2013). Professionals such as paediatricians and/or educational psychologists must be involved in assessing whether this criterion has been met.

It is easy when assessing the resources of a child to concentrate on what the child needs, i.e. the problems they encounter. This may be done for good reasons but, of course, it is not the total picture. Each child is unique and brings to a given environmental context resources that may involve strengths as well as weaknesses. These strengths may take the form of personal qualities, such as high motivation or resilience (e.g. the ability to come back after failure). This is a splendid resource to have and ultimately will have an effect on the outcome, if appropriately utilized. High motivation and the ability to persevere with a task are other beneficial qualities. We know that in two children with similar attributes, the one with higher motivation, higher sustained attention and greater resilience will have a more favourable outcome.

In summary, the resources of the child are collected and assembled from a variety of sources. They are not reliant on one or two tests but involve both quantitative and qualitative information that together build up a profile of the child. It is not simply 'testing' the child. This is the first arm of our triad of parameters that eventually build up the total picture of the ecosystem in which the child is operating. Finally, and of crucial importance, any summary of the individual is not complete without listing the strengths a child may possess. Using the strengths in situations that can improve other skills will make support and intervention much easier. All this information is collated for the planning of a support programme.

## Collecting information on the environmental context

The second arm of our triad of parameters involves the context in which the child is operating. It is not our aim to evaluate these parameters but to describe them so that we can understand the support that may be available. We have divided these contextual parameters into home, school, health and community.

*The home*

The main point to remember about the home context is that the parents will most prob-ably want and need to be *empowered*. It is no longer acceptable that so-called 'experts' come in to advise on what should be done. There needs to be a genuine partnership between the parents, the home context and the movement coach/named person, who together can devise the most appropriate course of action for the child. This could involve the parents working with the child in different ways, which we describe in Chapter 7. What is being explored here are the possibilities for a partnership, with parents being empowered to take charge of any support that is given in the home. The collection of information must be conducted with sensitivity and with the parents taking the lead on the options that may emerge from talks with different professionals and the movement coach/named person. It may be that some parents offer their cooperation in a structured programme. Others may simply want a set of ideas to work on while others may want or need only general guidelines. Some may feel that the child's needs are being addressed enough in other arenas. It is the parents' choice, aided by information from others to empower that choice (Bernheimer and Keogh 1995; Beveridge 2005).

In this vein, we support the approach of the Canadian group who have called their model *Partnering for Change* (P4C) (Missiuna et al. 2011). Their approach involves a partnership between therapists, parents and educators to create environments that will facilitate successful participation for all students. They collaboratively design environments that foster motor-skill development in children of all abilities, differ-entiate instruction for children who are experiencing challenges and accommodate students who need to participate in a different way. All involved parties contribute their skills to all pupils across the needs of the children. This approach is discussed in more detail in Chapters 6 and 8.

*The school*

In many countries, schools have a policy for what is often called special educational needs. This may involve a leader or coordinator who is responsible for organizing the support a particular child may need. If a school is part of a school district or local authority, their policies of funding and support will influence the organization of any support in the school. Therefore, the first port of call in a primary school will be the class teacher followed by the special needs coordinator (SENCO), if there is one. In the secondary school it will be the SENCO because the pupil moves from class to class and subject to subject.

Questions that could be asked include whether movement difficulties have been recog-nized within the overall framework of special needs? Is there any support from within the school, such as from the physical education and/or science/craft departments? Do teachers or teaching assistants have any training in the area of motor development? Is any in-class support provided or is the child withdrawn from the class for special tuition? Has the school made any recommendations for activities and support that can be done at home? Is there any peripatetic support from occupational or physical therapists?

It is recognized that any support within the school will depend upon both local and national policies on disability in general and motor difficulties in particular. The collection of information from the school and education system is an important feature when building the overall profile of what support might be available.

### The health services

The health service has always been a major player in providing support of various kinds to children with movement difficulties. Occupational therapist and physiotherapists have specific expertise in this area and are a good source of advice and support. However, it is rare to find a health service that provides therapists to work with children showing movement difficulties on an ongoing, week-by-week basis. What is required when collecting information from the health services is to ascertain what is available, who is available and where they work, i.e. in schools, home, a developmental centre or a combination of the above. Do the professionals work with individual children or in groups? How often do the health professionals see a child, either at home or in schools? When they do see the child themselves are they amenable to providing guidelines that can be used by others? It has been well established that teachers and parents can work effectively with children showing movement difficulties when they are given appropriate guidance by professionals (Sugden and Chambers 2003).

### The community

A final cornerstone of support, that is often lacking or unknown, is support that is available in the community. This can be in community centres, where groups of parents and children with movement difficulties can meet and engage in practical activities or simply exchange ideas. Also, sports centres that actively seek out children with various forms of movement difficulty to engage in their activities. There is a difference between a sports centre that simply welcomes children with difficulties to one that actively tries to recruit them, thereby extending the diversity of children they cater for and from which all children can benefit. Again, it is information of this kind that is of great utility to the named person/movement coach when they are building the profile of the child and his or her environment (see Box 4.4).

| Box 4.4 Environmental variables for participation | |
|---|---|
| School | Policies; practices; SENCO |
| Home | Family activities; parents |
| Community | Community sport; access; sports centres; parent groups |

## Case studies

In the final sections of this chapter we present various case studies as examples of the kinds of children who may be seen and the types of environmental context in which they are situated with different possibilities for support. These case studies will be used in subsequent chapters to illustrate how we move from collecting information to the various types of support and/or intervention that are offered.

## Three case studies from developmental coordination disorder

*Adam*

Adam is a 9-year-old boy of average ability in literacy and numeracy but who has struggled with his motor skills since he was a toddler. He had a typical term birth and process but was delayed in many of his motor milestones. He was 9 months of age before he could roll from back to stomach and 16 months before he could walk unaided. His fine motor development was also delayed. He was 7–8 months before he could reach for an object and around 13–14 months before he could make a neat pincer grip. He is the second child in the household having a younger sister who developed in a typical manner. His parents noticed his delays but were not overly concerned until he went to school. At school the delay seemed to be holding him back in some manual activities, handwriting and in physical education, where his teacher reported that he was clumsy and awkward compared to other children.

Adam is a cheerful and amiable young boy, with friends with whom he engages in recreational activities, such as football and other games out of school. However, his friends are now noticing his difficulties and are engaging in some good-natured teasing. Adam takes these in his stride at the present time, but his parents and teachers are becoming a little concerned that this may become more difficult for him and affect his friendship group. The situation is now a little more serious as he cannot ride a bicycle, whereas his friends are using their bikes to go to the park and for other recreational areas. In the classroom, his writing is very slow and when he does speed up it becomes illegible. In addition, he becomes easily confused when asked to perform a sequence of tasks, such as packing his bag or lunch box for school.

Until recently, these issues were not too problematic and, outwardly, Adam did not seem unduly concerned by them. However, of late he has started to mention the cycling and writing in class and his parents and teachers are keen that some form of support is given so that he can keep engaging in play activities with his friends and can adequately deal with his writing difficulties in the classroom. Adam pays attention in class and has no real behavioural difficulties.

It was agreed by Adam's parents and teachers that, with his cooperation, there should be a more formal assessment of his motor skills and the local health authority was asked to do this. In the first instance, the occupational therapist talked to his teacher and parents and to Adam, and as a first step asked the teacher and parents to complete an MABC-2 Checklist. As noted earlier in the chapter, this has three sections with the first two looking at motor skill performance and the third noting any behaviours that influence his motor skills. Overall, on Adam scored 16 in sections A and B, which put him in the 5th to 15th centile range, meaning that his skills will need to be monitored for further progress. However, his profile was uneven in these sections. In Section A, which assesses those skills where the environment is stable and predictable, he was good on self-care and some classroom skills but poor on other classroom skills such as manipulating, drawing and writing, and equally poor on physical education and recreational skills. In section B, where the environment is moving or unpredictable, he scored poorly. His overall score of around the 8th to 10th centile was aided by his competence at self-care skills of various activities in dressing, whereas in all other aspects he was in the lowest 5%. In Section C, which looks at non-motor factors that may affect movement, he scored a 'yes' for hesitant, forgetful and disorganized but was mostly typical in all the other items. However, teachers noted that he was starting to become upset by failure and tended to underestimate his abilities. There was some divergence of opinion between parents and teachers in their reports, but this was mainly because parents did not observe all the activities mentioned by the teachers but, in the main, they were in concordance with each other.

Following this, the occupational therapist conducted a formal MABC-2 Test assessment. The test, as noted in the early part of the chapter, has three sections to it with two or three items in each component part. Overall, Adam had a score of 44, which put him at the 2nd centile, indicating that his movement difficulties would require immediate attention. His scores across the three components were not similar, with real movement difficulties in the manual dexterity and balance components. In the manual dexterity section he scored 14, which is at the 2nd centile; in balance he scored 14, which also is at the 2nd centile; while in the aiming and catching section he scored 16, which is at the 25th centile.

The MABC-2 Test and Checklist results are important indicators of the difficulties, and indeed some of the strengths, that Adam possesses. If we were testing for a diagnosis of DCD, then the test score of the lowest 2% would go some way to satisfying Criterion A in the DSM-5, indicating a significant impairment of movement. as measured by a culturally appropriate standardized test. Similarly, a score in the lowest 5% on the MABC Checklist would go part of the way to meeting Criterion B of the DSM-5, indicating that the impairment noted in Criterion A has a detrimental effect on activities of everyday living. However, it must be stated again that neither the MABC-2 nor any other test of its type can diagnose DCD. The diagnosis must be made by suitably qualified and experienced professionals, such as a paediatrician or educational psychologist, based

> **Box 4.5** Summary Adam (9y)
>
> ✓ History of motor delay
> ✓ Difficulties in manual skills, slow writing and untidy when faster
> ✓ Physical education is now challenging
> ✓ Amiable with friends and but recently shown anxieties
> ✓ Poor bike-riding and ball skills
> ✓ Formal assessment on the MABC-2: Test lowest 2%; Checklist 5%–15%
> ✓ Possible DCD

on all the information presented to them. Thus, for an official diagnosis of DCD to be given, all four criteria from DSM-5 would need to be satisfied. For that to occur Criterion D, which involves exclusionary clauses, must be addressed. A paediatrician and/or an educational psychologist would examine Adam and note that he does not have CP or any other neurological disorder that could produce similar symptoms. Also, that any difficulties he has are over and above those that would be expected from his overall ability/intelligence.

Finally, Adam was given the DASH test (Barnett et al. 2017) and on the five subtests was scored in the lowest 5% for speed, thus confirming the informal observations from the teacher.

*Jenny*
Jenny is a 13-year-old girl, quiet and reserved who has had a history of what could be called neuromotor difficulties. She was born at 25 weeks' gestation weighing 2lbs 10oz. She has been delayed in all her motor skills: rolling, sitting, standing and walking. In her first year of life she was assessed for suspected CP because she presented hypertonicity in her arms, but this seemed to disappear, and no diagnosis of CP was ever given. She was delayed in her speech and has had numerous assessments for this. These have concluded that she has no problem with either expressive or receptive language in terms of either semantics or syntax, but she does have an articulation difficulty, which she now finds embarrassing. She has had speech therapy over the years.

Jenny is highly intelligent. Although no formal IQ tests have been given, on school-related tests in numeracy, literacy and other parts of the curriculum she scores highest in her year. Teachers report that she is one of the brightest children they have ever seen. From the age of 4 she could read and by 7 was reading at the level of a 12-year-old level. Her written compositions are detailed and imaginative, with many of them published in the school magazine; she has won local writing competitions. Similarly, in mathematics, she is working on problems way beyond her age and will be taking A-level mathematics (a national examination normally taken by 17/18-year-olds). This picture of academic excellence is seen across the curriculum except in areas where controlled movements are required. Thus, in physical education she is 'awkward' and 'clumsy' and does not engage in physical activities out of school. In home economics classes she is careful and meticulous but very slow and the same applies to her work in the science laboratory. In most lessons writing is becoming an issue as her lessons now demand quicker, legible writing. She can write very neatly but it is very slow. In addition, her keyboard skills are also poor, and even though there is a keyboard class offered after school, her two friends do not attend and so Jenny is reluctant to go on her own for fear of ridicule.

Socially, Jenny is reserved and is not a great mixer in her peer group. This is starting to become an issue with her as she is at an age when young adolescents are starting to become more independent and moving in groups of like-minded young people. However, she does have two close girlfriends. They have been together since early in primary school and the three of them seem to be mutually supportive; her friends do help her mix with the peer group. There are activities that are becoming an issue for Jenny for example, she cannot ride a bicycle. Her two friends are quite athletic and they ride much of the time. She is also awkward in situations where there is dancing and music as she is poorly coordinated and, in her words, 'gawky'. Jenny is kind and considerate and is an animal lover, spending time at weekends at a local donkey sanctuary. She finds this activity worthwhile and gets much out of it but it reinforces her social isolation from her peer group. She has a mobile phone, but it is noticeable that in peer company she uses it for calling rather than texting, like the other girls of her age.

When discussing her situation, Jenny is frank and to the point, saying what she is good at and where she needs support. She says she does want help and would like some guidance as to what to do.

As with Adam, a first port of call after discussions with teachers and parents was some form of formal assessment. While recognizing this may not provide any new information it would confirm what is already known. Both the MABC-2 Checklist and Test were given and, as expected, Jenny scored in the lowest 1% in both. There were, however, some notable scores. On the Checklist, she stated 'yes' only to underestimating her ability, being timid and becoming anxious; in all other behaviours she stated 'no', This is a bonus when it comes to building a profile for Jenny and examining her strengths; it can be used to support her needs in the movement area. As we often say an individual with a movement difficulty and no organization problems, is very different to one who has both; the outcome for the former may be much more positive. On the manual skills part of the Test, Jenny was extremely accurate in everything she did, but the speed at

> **Box 4.6** Summary Jenny (13y)
>
> Preterm birth and low birthweight
> Speech difficulty
> Very high IQ
> Poor handwriting and keyboard skills
> Quiet and reserved
> Has two very supportive friends, but lately not mixing as much as a result of poor motor skills
> Uses mobile to call rather than text
> Keen to improve
> Lowest 1% on the MABC-2

which she accomplished the tasks placed her in the lowest 1%. This also was her score on the balance activities. The aiming and catching were a little better, mainly due to her being able to take her time throwing at a target. As with Adam, for a diagnosis of DCD to be given, Jenny would need to be seen by a paediatrician and/or educational psychologist to exclude CP (this had been done earlier in her life) and to show that her difficulties in the motor area were over and above those that would be expected from her overall intelligence.

On the DASH test (Barnett et al. 2006, 2010) Jenny mirrored the slow manual skills scores from the MABC Test, scoring in the lowest 1% for her age group. This percentage was roughly the same across all five subtests of the DASH.

Jenny is very keen to improve. As we can see in her profile and objectives, she is clear about what she wants to achieve and is looking for guidance as to how to do this. The plan is to organize the support structure such that it is built into the activities of her daily life and is supported by different individuals in different contexts. This will involve her two friends and advice and help from health and educational professionals.

*James*

James is 20 years of age and in his first year at university studying chemistry. He has chosen to go to a university away from his home and so is living in student accommodation. A studious young man, James has a history of movement difficulties. These have troubled him all the way through school and at age 9 years he had a diagnosis of DCD. This diagnosis was conducted in an appropriate manner and fulfilled all the criteria from DSM IV-TR (APA 2002), which were the prevailing criteria at the time.

The collection of information on James started with his parents providing both a verbal and written report of his movement difficulties. These had been noticeable since he was a toddler when he was delayed in most motor milestones. He did not walk until he was 16 months old, was late in activities such as jumping and had great difficulty even at 9 years with hopping, particularly when asked to hop to a rhythm. He was poor at ball games and did not like physical education because he was always regarded as one of the worst at games in his year. His fine motor abilities appeared to be good and his handwriting was neat, although quite slow. His teachers also reported that in gross motor activities he was poor, but his fine motor abilities were good. He was assessed by an occupational therapist and an educational psychologist and seen by a paediatrician.

The occupational therapist administered the MABC-1 (Henderson and Sugden 1992) to James, obtaining checklist scores from both parents and teachers. The MABC Test was given and the results showed James to have quite severe difficulties in the areas of aiming and catching and balance. He was able to adjust appropriately when the environment was moving or unpredictable in nearly all items of self-care and classroom skills, ball skills and recreational and physical education skills. On both the test and the checklist he was in the typical range on practically all areas of fine motor demands. Thus, his writing was fine, if a little slow; he could use scissors, manipulate small objects and dress himself. Both test and checklist results placed him in the 30th to 40th centile on these items. In balance and aiming and catching he was in the lowest 2%. Overall, he was in the 5th to 15th centile, which would be in the monitoring range rather than requiring immediate action. The occupational therapist thought that his catching, balance, and recreational skills were poor enough for her to recommend that Criteria A and B of DSM-IV were satisfied. The educational psychologist tested James for intelligence on an individually administered test and he scored 136, with little discrepancy between verbal and performance scores. This is over 2 standard deviations above the mean of 100 and puts him well into the top 2% of the population. Reports from his teacher noted that he was achieving at this level in his academic work. Accordingly, it was obvious that lack of intelligence was not a factor in his poor motor skills. At the age of 9 years, the paediatrician had no hesitation from the information gleaned in giving a diagnosis of DCD. Unfortunately, as we will see later, this diagnosis did not bring any extra help or support from either health or education authorities.

Other factors to note about James are that as a child he was quite distressed about his poor skills, particularly in the physical education classes. This continued to worry him into his teens. However, although he was awkward and clumsy, and indeed had an ungainly gait when running, he could run very well in long-distance events. He found that he had excellent stamina and ran in the school cross-country team and enjoyed this activity as it kept him fit and healthy and gave him social standing. He still worried about his lack of coordination however, especially because, no matter

> **Box 4.7** Summary James (20y)
>
> Early history and continuing movement problems
>
> Manual skills good but lowest on 5% on gross and manual and balance and agility on MABC-1 Test and Checklist
>
> Ungainly runner, but good endurance in cross-country participation
>
> Poor bike riding which is restricting friendships
>
> Pragmatic about difficulties, but university offers a fresh start
>
> Unable to drive, which may affect social situations

how much he tried (as he reported), he could not ride a bicycle. His cross-country running became his sole social activity, but his main friends from school were not part of that group. His friends did a lot of cycling, often spending an entire day on their bikes where they would ride 30 to 40 miles and have various refreshment stops. This social activity was not available to James as he had given up on learning to ride a bicycle when he was around 12 years of age and at 16 felt he could not take it up again. At 17 when all his friends were learning to drive, James opted out and did not even attempt it. As he now approaches university life, he knows he may be able to join a running group, but he cannot ride a bicycle, is still awkward and ungainly and has never tried to drive a car.

James, although a little concerned about this, is also phlegmatic about the whole situation. However, he is starting to wonder whether there will be any support that may help him pick up the skills he is lacking in a socially acceptable manner, without embarrassment. Moving away to university may be chance for him to do this and he is looking for some options as to the next step.

## Examples from children with other developmental disorders

In Chapter 1 we described how children with movement difficulties could be placed broadly into two categories: those with movement difficulties as a primary defining condition such as the three we have described above and those who have another primary defining condition, but also have movement difficulties as secondary characteristics. The following children fit into this latter category.

### Marie

Marie is a 12-year-old girl just starting her first year of secondary school. During her primary school years she was diagnosed with attention-deficit disorder (ADD), primarily because of her attention difficulties that were evidenced without any accompanying hyperactivity. The attention difficulties were first seen when Marie was in preschool when teachers noticed that she often drifted and, to use their words, appeared 'vacant'. As she was young for her year, being a June birth, the teachers initially regarded this as immaturity. However, this continued through primary school and, indeed, became more pronounced. It involved forgetting to give parents messages and notes about parents evening; being late from break and dinner for no apparent reason; leaving school essentials, such as pencils and books, at home or not bringing them home when needed. It was in the classroom, however, that there was the greatest concern. The lack of attention/daydreaming took a number of forms. First, Marie had problems coming to attention and she often missed what the main point of a topic or indeed a lesson was. When she did come to attention, she often concentrated on the wrong point of any story or debate or what was required in an assignment. Third, when she did pay attention to the correct topic it was often only a short time before she drifted again into her 'own world'. The diagnosis of ADD was given according to DSM-IV, with more than six of the diagnostic characteristics listed in criteria A1. An example of these are A1b 'often has difficulty sustaining attention in tasks or play activities'; A1c, 'often does not seem to listen when spoken to directly' and A1i: 'is often forgetful in daily activities' (APA 2002).

In all, Marie satisfied seven of the nine characteristics listed under criteria A1. She exhibited one or two characteristics under the hyperactivity section of criteria A2, but not enough for a diagnosis of ADHD to be given. Her parents and teachers were given the Connors Checklist to complete and, again, the low attention scores were noted. The Connors Checklist has two versions, with the long versions often used for initial evaluations when ADHD is suspected. The short version can be used to measure hyperactivity over time in children and adolescents. It can help to provide clinical information to support decisions about classification that will guide support and intervention.

A diagnosis of ADD was given as the symptoms were present early in life and are present both at home and at school. In addition, the symptoms interfere with her social and academic life and are not due to any other mental disorder.

Marie's ability in most subjects was below the mean of her peers, scoring around the 25th centile in most subjects; however, it was not low enough for her to receive any extra help in class, other than that provided by her teacher when she differentiates the lesson content from the set assignments.

As she grew up problems started to appear more at home. Her parents reported that she daydreamed a lot and missed requests or instructions. When out she often forgot to phone home to reassure parents where she was. This concerned her parents as she was starting to socialize outside of school. Marie is a quiet and reserved young girl and is generally regarded as being 'nice' by peers.

**Box 4.8** Marie (12y)

ADD diagnosis

Low average overall ability (25th centile)

Poor motor skills, including self-care skills

Low achiever, sets low targets, low self-esteem and upset by failure

Quiet, reserved and 'nice'

Participation seen as the issue from start

Her gross motor skills have been poor throughout her childhood, perhaps because she hardly participated in any activities in or out of school. She never tried to ride a bicycle and she did not take part in any recreational activities. Her fine motor skills were also poor. She was clumsy when using scissors and had untidy handwriting. She was slow to dress in the mornings, being easily distracted, and often missed school buses. When she did engage in motor activities, she was timid and fearful, even in non-threatening situations. She underestimated her ability, was upset by failure and set low goals. It is difficult to disentangle her poor motor skills from her ADD and other social and emotional characteristics. She has a low self-concept, which is not helped by her poor motor performance. The main cause for concern of her parents and teachers and Marie herself is her lack of participation; she actively avoids any participation because of her embarrassment. Thus, all parties agree that for Marie to improve her motor skills she needs to participate more. All agree that the motor skills she learns may be used to improve her attention and learning overall. As we said earlier, movement can serve two functions: first one can *learn a* motor skills, that is learning to move, or one can use movement as a vehicle to learn other skills, moving to learn.

*Andrew*

Andrew is a 9-year-old boy who has been diagnosed with high-functioning autism. He was diagnosed at the age of 5 as having Asperger syndrome under the DSM-IV (APA 2002) criteria. But as noted in Chapter 1, in the DSM-5 Asperger syndrome is classified under the general autistic spectrum disorder (APA 2013). Under this most recent classification Andrew fulfills all the criteria in sections A to E. In category A, he clearly has deficits in social communication and social interaction across several environmental contexts and he has repetitive restricted patterns of behaviour as listed in criterion B. These behaviours have been noticed from an early age and led to him being disadvantaged in social and school situations. They are not better explained by other factors, such as a general delay or intellectual disability.

Observations that gave rise to concern started when Andrew was a toddler. His parents have an older son and naturally made comparisons. The first signs were at around

18 months of age when the perceived lack of interaction with his parents and older brother seemed to become more prominent. Andrew did have words at that age but used them rather haphazardly and often not in the appropriate context. He also engaged in echolalia. At 2 to 3 years of age this lack of appropriate use of language became more pronounced. Equally worrying was his impoverished engagement in other forms of communication, such as eye contact and hugging and touching. He had a hard time with reciprocal interactions, finding it difficult to engage appropriately with his parents or brother and others. At 4 to 5 years of age his speech became more idiosyncratic. It was syntactically good and quite sophisticated, and the semantics were also of a high standard; however, the context in which these were used was highly inappropriate. The language, although quite sophisticated for his age, was rarely in synchrony with the social situation he was in. The communication was usually one sided, with him speaking but not interacting. Explanations for this, as noted in chapter 1, could include an impoverished theory of mind, an impairment of empathy, or not recognizing the social context in which he and others are situated.

In addition to the social and use of language impairments, Andrew also displayed a range of other behaviours that gave rise to the early diagnosis of Asperger syndrome. At an early age he engaged in simple stereotypical behaviours, such as lining up objects and holding objects close to his eyes and staring at them. At 4 to 5 years of age he became very resistant to change, as evidenced by sticking to routines in a rigid manner and having strict food preferences. In addition, he had a paradoxical sensitivity, or lack of it, to smells, noises, textures, and other sensory stimuli. He would develop a fascination with an object for a time and then become absorbed with another object. These objects have included clocks, simple musical tunes and decorative plates kept in the house. With age, his routines have become more rigid with respect to washing, toileting and dressing in a strict order. His parents have been excellent in understanding these behaviours and have attempted to accommodate them. At preschool, Andrew's behaviour was also accommodated in a pleasing manner.

When he moved on to primary school the staff were aware of his needs and provided some part-time assistance, paid for by the local education authority.

Andrew is very bright. He could read quite fluently by the age of 5 and his numeracy scores place him in the top 5% of his age group. However, these are done with little meaning to the context. He can answer comprehension questions on a text he has read and although his answers clearly show that he has read it and understood the text, the answers often reflect his own peculiar take on a story. Now, at 9 years of age he no longer throws tantrums as he did when he was younger and things did not go his way. But he does become isolated and refuses to interact with the teachers, parents, or his peers when he feels that his wants and needs are not being met to his satisfaction.

> **Box 4.9** Andrew (9y)
>
> High functioning autism
> History of inappropriate language – wrong context for topic
> Bullied about his awkwardness, gait and lack of motor ability
> Stubborn and can refuse to interact
> Discusses all this self-referenced

Alongside all of this, he has motor difficulties, which may seem minor by comparison to his other needs, but they are now becoming a source of stress for him. Until the last couple of years, his classmates have tolerated and indeed helped him in his autistic tendencies. This has continued in class but in the playground, in physical education lessons and in social situations outside of school, he has become the object of ridicule to some of his peers. This is because he is terribly clumsy with a gait that is so awkward that it looks as if a different motor is driving each of his limbs independently. He cannot ride a bicycle. All these cause him distress and make him more isolated, both in and outside of school. He has few friends and his lack of participation in leisure activities only serves to heighten his isolated, autistic behaviour. He has had no formal motor skill diagnosis.

When Andrew discusses all this he does it solely from his viewpoint and does recognize that others may be able to help him. His parents and teachers feel a new approach is required as he enters the last year of primary school so that he can acquire a new and additional set of behaviours that will help him cope in the much bigger, and perhaps threatening, world of secondary school. Any support that is planned for his movement difficulties must be in synchrony with his autistic needs and *moving to learn* may be an appropriate way forward.

### Paul

Our final case is Paul who is a 14-year-old boy in a mainstream secondary school. Paul is an example we often see in our schools in that he has no specified diagnosis for any condition. He does not stand out in any one area of disability, yet overall he is a worry to parents and teachers as he underachieves in several areas, which affects this self-esteem, self-concept and friendships in and out of school.

From an early age, Paul's parents, who have three other children, noticed that Paul was different. He was delayed in his motor skills, language and other forms of communication and generally did not seem as inquisitive as his siblings. His speech continued to be delayed and, although he can now communicate adequately, he does have a speech impediment that makes fast responses difficult. As a toddler and young child, he was content to play on his own, generally with the same toys. After a long period he would switch to another set of toys and play with them for a similarly long period. He did not interact much with his peers in preschool and this continued throughout his primary school. He was slow in learning to read and read at a level 2 years below his chronological age. His numeracy was the same, not being entirely poor at this subject, but showing a number of problems in areas that most children readily pick up. He took a long time to learn some of the basics, which in turn prevented him from keeping up with his peers when they used the basic skills to solve such challenges as word problems.

His motor skills have always been poor. He has had no support for these, as it seems they were considered by his parents and teachers to be of a lower priority than his other needs. We noted above his delay in walking and this delay was evident with most of his fundamental motor skills. We have often noted that by 6 to 7 years of age, a typically developing child will have all the naturally developing motor skills they ever attain in life. By then they can walk, run, jump, hop, skip, throw, catch, climb, write, draw, copy, manipulate reach and grasp, etc. Beyond this age, these skills are refined to be used in different contexts and adapted to the many demands of daily living. Paul was deficient in many of these skills, never outstandingly bad in any one, but showing delays of some kind in all of them.

Paul is keen to learn most things at the present time but he is now starting to avoid situations in which he will either fail of be shown to take much longer to learn than his friends. He does have some friends, as he is a likeable boy. He has been tested in several areas and found to be, on average, around the 15th to 20th centile. This would include overall ability, with an IQ of 82 at 9 years of age. A motor test (not named) placed him at the 20th centile and his in-class work placed him at roughly the same level.

Thus, we have a boy who has no formal diagnosis of any disorder and no formal learning difficulty, neither general nor specific. He is, however, generally behind in numeracy and literacy. He has no diagnosis of a motor difficulty, although there are clearly concerns in this area. Although Paul is showing some perseveration difficulties, these are not enough for a diagnosis of ASD. He has attention difficulties when he is asked to do things he does not appear interested in. He has movement difficulties, but again, not enough to have attracted extra support.

In short, Paul is the type of boy we often see in our schools with no diagnosis of a specific condition but enough general difficulties to warrant support. Paul is now at the stage where he is watching other children overtake him in most areas. He is smart enough to recognize that he has some difficulties and he is becoming concerned about losing the friendships he has kept over the years. He is now in a 'big' secondary school where he

---

**Box 4.10** Paul (14y)

Underachieves across the board

Low self-concept and self-esteem

Delayed language and reading

General poor motor skills

Around 20th centile in most areas, including motor skills

Concerned about friendships; becoming morose

---

can get lost and his self-concept and self-esteem are beginning to fall. He is becoming a little morose and inward looking.

The way forward for Paul is complex and will involve a group of support persons working together in a coordinated manner, with Paul's approval, to address some of these issues. Learning motor skills can play a role here but only as part of an overall approach addressing multiple issues.

## Comments on the case studies

The preceding six case studies have illustrated diversity in the children and young people we see with movement difficulties in homes at school and in the community. The sex ratio, four males to two females, is a roughly the same as we see.

A point to emphasize here is that these individuals all show motor problems to some degree, but these are embedded in a complexity of other issues such as personal resources and the environmental context. This is why we develop programmes tailored to these individual situations.

## Summary

The collation of information to plan a programme of support is a multifaceted task. It is not simply assessing the child using a checklist or standardized test; these will provide some valuable information but clearly not all. It is the individual in both the broad and narrow context and how these multiple inputs converge to provide the complete information that will lead to an effective support for programme. It is, in short, a collection of information from the total ecological setting. Thus, we have outlined the types of information that can be collected on the individual, ranging from commercial tests to professional and clinical observations and from families and friends who can provide equally valid insights into the individual's strengths and weaknesses. We believe that it is only this comprehensive collection of information from multiple sources that can create successful intervention and support.

From this collection of information, the interested parties come together to produce a profile of the child and from which are generated a set of objectives and their priorities. This is a team effort, with any support being multilayered and different individuals having an input, but never forgetting the child's interests and choices are at the heart of the exercise.

## References

APA (2000) *Diagnostic and Statistical Manual of Mental Disorders,* 4th edition (DSM-IV). Washington DC: American Psychiatric Association.

APA (2013) *Diagnostic and Statistical Manual of Mental Disorders,* 5th edition (DSM-5). Washington DC: American Psychiatric Association.

Barnett A, Henderson SE, Scheib B, Schulz J (2007) *Detailed Assessment of Speed of Handwriting (DASH).* London: Pearson.

Barnett AL, Henderson SE, Scheib B, Schulz J (2011) Handwriting difficulties and their assessment in young adults with DCD: Extension of the DASH for 17-25-year-olds. *J Adult Dev* 18: 114–121.

Barnett A, Henderson SE, Scheib B, Schulz J (2009) Development and standardization of a new handwriting speed test: the DASH. *Brit J Educ Psychol Mon Series II* 6: 137–157.

Bernheimer LP, Keogh BK (1995) Weaving interventions into the fabric of everyday life: an approach to family assessment. *Topics Early Child Spec Educ* 15: 415–433.

Beveridge S (2005) *Children, Families and Schools. Developing Partnerships for Education.* London: Routledge Falmer.

Blank R, Barnett AL, Cairney J, et al. (2019) International clinical practice recommendations on the definition, diagnosis, assessment, intervention, and psychosocial aspects of developmental coordination disorder. *Dev Med Child Neurol* 61: 242–285.

Bruninks RH, Bruininks BD (2007) *Bruininks-Oseretsky Test of Motor Performance,* 2nd edition. Minneapolis, MN: American Guidance Service.

Chambers ME, Sugden DA (2002) The identification and assessment of young children with movement difficulties. *Int Early Years Educ* 10: 157–176.

Chambers ME, Sugden DA (2006) *Early Years Movement Skills: Description, Diagnosis and Intervention.* London: John Wiley and Sons.

Henderson SE, Sugden DA, Barnett A (2007) *Movement Assessment Battery for Children,* 2nd edition. Pearson: London.

Kirby A, Sugden DA, Beveridge SE, Edwards L, Edwards R (2008a) Dyslexia and developmental coordination disorder in further and higher education. *Dyslexia* 14: 197–213.

Kirby A, Sugden D, Beveridge S, Edwards L (2008) Developmental co-ordination disorder (DCD) in adults and adolescents. *J Res Spec Educ Needs* 8: 120–131.

Kirby A, Edwards L, Sugden DA, Rosenbaum S (2010) The development and standardization of the Adult Developmental Co-ordination Disorders/Dyspraxia Checklist (ADC). *Res Dev Disabil* 31: 131–139.

Kirby A, Edwards L, Sugden DA (2011) Emerging adulthood in developmental coordination disorder: parent and young adult perspectives. *Res Dev Disabil* 32: 135–160.

Missiuna C, Pollock N, Campbell W, Levac D, Whalen S (2011) *CanChild Partnering for Change?* Hamilton ON: McMaster University.

Missiuna C, Pollock N, Law M (2004) *Perceived Efficacy of Goal Setting in Young Children (PEGS).* San Antonio, TX: Psychological Corporation.

Rihtman T, Wilson BN, Parush S (2011) Development of the Little Developmental Coordination Disorder Questionnaire for Preschoolers and preliminary evidence of its psychometric properties in Israel. *Res Dev Disabil* 32: 1378–1387.

Schoemaker MM, Wilson B (2015) Screening for developmental coordination disorder in children. In Cairney J (ed.). *Secondary Consequences of Developmental Coordination Disorder.* Toronto ON: University of Toronto Press, pp. 169–191.

Schoemaker MM, Niemeir AS, Flapper BCT, Smits-Engelsman BCM (2012) Validity and reliability of the Movement Assessment Battery for Children-2 Checklist for children with and without motor impairments. *Dev Med Child Neurol* 54: 368–375.

Schoemaker MM, Smits-Engelsman B, Jongmans MJ (2003) Psychometric properties of the Movement Assessment Battery for Children Checklist as a screening instrument for children with developmental coordination disorder. *Br J Educ Psychol* 73: 425–441.

Schultz J, Henderson SE, Sugden DA, Barnet AL (2011) Structural validity of the MABC Test: factor structure comparisons across three age groups. *Res Dev Disabil* 32: 1361–1369.

Sugden DA, Chambers ME (2003) Intervention in children with DCD: the role of parents and teachers. *Br J Educ Psychol* 73: 545–561.

Sugden DA, Henderson SE (2007) *Ecological Intervention for Children with Movement Difficulties.* Pearson: London.

Ulrich D (2000) *Test of Gross Motor Development-2.* Austin Texas: Pro-Ed.

Wilson PH, Kaplan BJ, Crawford SG, Roberts G (2007) *The Developmental Coordination Disorder Questionnaire 2007.* Calgary, Canada: Alberta Children's Hospital Decision Support Research Team.

Wilson BN, Kaplan KJ, Crawford SG, Campbell A, Dewey D (2000) Reliability and validity of a parent questionnaire on childhood motor skills. *Am J Occup Ther* 54: 484–493.

Wilson BN, Creighton D, Crawford SG, et al. (2014). Psychometric properties of the Canadian Little Developmental Coordination Disorder Questionnaire for Preschool Children. *Phys Occup Ther Pediatr* 35: 116–131.

# Chapter 5

## From profiles through objectives to action

In Chapter 4 we showed how the child's profile is a summary of the information collected from various sources. The same child may act differently in different contexts and change over time, so the profile must take account of this. It is not just the resources of the child that feed into the profiling, but the influencing constraints, which will affect any goals, objectives and plans.

When examining the profiles, we try to note the variables that influence the child's daily functioning. These include areas that the individuals concerned feel are necessary to work on, as well as the strengths of the child that will complement any external support and intervention.

A child with a motor problem and an attention difficulty will require a different approach to one who can pay full attention and is motivated. Similarly, a child who seems to be downhearted with his or her failed attempts at tasks will require a different approach to one who 'bounces' back after failure.

## Participation and learning

A major part of the process of creating a profile for a child or young person is to examine the balance between **participation level** and **learning**. Participation level is a crucial factor in the learning process, with many variables outside of the child's control that affect how much he or she can participate. Part of the profiling process is to see where

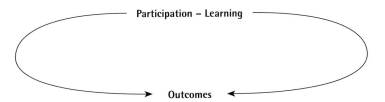

**Figure 5.1** Participation and learning.

the emphasis between participation and learning needs to be placed. For example, if a 6-year-old child has a movement problem but has had restricted opportunities for movement activities, whether at home, school or in the community, then participation would be something to look at in the first instance. Conversely, if the child has been actively engaged in activities but is still having movement difficulties, then the activities that are being taught and how they are presented in teaching, therapeutic, or daily life situations, needs to be examined at. Figure 5.1 shows the relationship between participation and learning.

*Participation*
Participation is one of the categories of the International Classification of Functioning, Disability and Health (ICF) model (WHO 2001). The others are body functions and structures; activities of people; and environmental factors.

This ICF model is similar to the one presented in this text that employs the variables of child or personal resources, environmental context and task choice and presentation. Participation is a feature of the environmental context. It is about including all people in all areas of life and some of the facilitators and barriers that can either help or hinder it. Figure 5.2 shows the multifaceted nature of participation and how it can be divided into steps to assist in the areas of **accessibility, appropriateness and meaningfulness**.

The first box in Figure 5.2 shows that the child should not have to work hard to be involved. The community, health services, schools and families can alter the context so that the child has easy access to participation. The second box shows that context needs to be appropriate to the child's needs with, for example, gross motor activities being available for the child who has difficulties in that area. The third box indicates

| The child needs to find it easy to be involved | The context needs to be appropriate to the child's needs | Context has to have meaning in the child's life |
|---|---|---|
| **Accessibility** | **Appropriateness** | **Meaningfulness** |

**Figure 5.2** The general and multiple components of participation.

that participation should be meaningful and motivating and not simply repetition of sets of exercises.

From work on children with developmental coordination disorder (DCD) we know that children with movement difficulties participate less than their peers, obtain less enjoyment from participation and that their families are not satisfied with the limited opportunities they are given. The effect of this is that individuals with movement difficulties have less time and fewer opportunities for learning motor skills, which can lead to secondary consequences such as reduced fitness, higher levels of fatty tissue, low self-concept and self-confidence and withdrawal from social situations (Cairney et al. 2010; Engel-Yeger and Kasis 2010; Magalhães et al. 2011). These negative outcomes are the same for children with other developmental disorders with movement difficulties. Indeed, these children would be more adversely affected because of their other difficulties.

Participation is not a unitary concept but can be within the community, or when more narrowly defined, within the learning situation itself (see Fig. 5.2). This is how learning and participation interact. In the first instance, at the broad level of participation the locus of control is usually outside of the control of family and the child, residing often in the local facilities available for the child. Such opportunities are often provided by community and sports centres. These centres need to be proactive in seeking out children with movement difficulties rather than having a passive, 'we welcome all' approach. This broad-based, community approach to participation would not only offer opportunities to help those that require it, but also increase the communities' awareness on the needs of all children. In this way, the objective of more time on task could be achieved through more opportunities being provided, thereby addressing the issue of accessibility (see Fig. 5.2).

A second way to look at participation and how it interacts with learning is in the support programmes themselves. These can range from formal sessions in a clinic, through more informal ones in the classroom, to small alterations to daily routines that can be seen in the home and elsewhere. Thus, when the individual is in a learning situation, at home, in school, or in the clinic setting, the aim is to achieve maximum participation on the task to be learned.

A real life situation of this is shown in a study by Chambers and Sugden (2014), who worked with preschool children showing movement difficulties. In this study, the persons providing the support were the teaching/learning assistants who worked with the children in their classrooms. Children were identified as having movement difficulties and three levels of participation and learning were employed in a continuous rather than discrete fashion, with the aim of a seamless progression from one level to the next. The approach was built upon the **'response to intervention'** model where the level of intervention is based upon how a child responds to a particular form of support (Chambers and Sugden 2014). In our study, we identified three levels of support that incorporated both participation and learning. The first of these we labelled **exposure.** This was simply to make available the activities that are usually present in daily life at school (but that could be incorporated in other contexts) if the child wished to choose them. Thus, activities for fine motor skills were available in the classroom for the child to choose, such as unimanual and bimanual manipulation, and reaching and grasping. In addition, gross motor activities such as agility and aiming and catching tasks were included. At this level the child chose whether or not to be engaged. Our second level was **experience.** Here the child was presented with an activity to work on and was encouraged to participate directly. No pressure was placed on the child and it involved no teaching or therapeutic work, but the level of engagement was greater than at the exposure level. The focus here was to give direct encouragement to the child to participate. The third level we called **direct teaching.** If the child showed little progress at the level of exposure and experience, then he or she would be taught the activity directly. If it was thought the activity was a useful or necessary part of the child's daily life, direct teaching would be desirable to equip the child with a necessary skill. Through this graded manner of presenting the various daily skills, both **participation** and **learning** are addressed in a fluid, seamless and flexible manner. This process will be elaborated on in Chapter 9. Figure 5.3 illustrates in more detail the kind of items that can enhance participation.

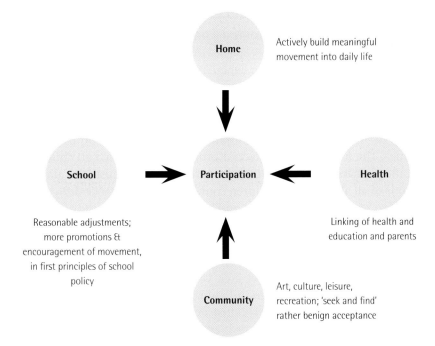

**Figure 5.3** Components of participation.

## Partnering for Change

This approach to participation is very much in line with the excellent work done in Canada led by Cheryl Missiuna and *CanChild*, the Partnering for Change (P4C) model (Missiuna et al. 2012, 2017). The P4C approach is a population health/community initiative where a team go into schools, not primarily to intervene but to observe, understand and provide some support for children with various difficulties, to prevent secondary consequences.

The goals of the P4C service delivery model are to

- facilitate earlier identification of students with special needs;
- build capacity of educators and parents to understand and manage children's needs;
- improve children's ability to participate in school and at home;
- facilitate self and family management to prevent secondary consequences (www.partneringforchange.ca).

P4C is a partnership between health and education, where occupational therapists go into schools one day a week and work with teachers. The work does not necessarily involve identifying a child and working on deficits, but is rather aimed at rearranging the environment and the context so that the child can achieve success in a natural manner. For example, adjusting the size of desks and chairs and sitting positions are small alterations that can be made to the context without the child having to follow detailed instructions. P4C is about building capacity through collaboration and coaching, in context. The context is the classroom, where the motor aspects of a task are analysed. For example, cutting shapes in mathematics, and how such a task can be modified to allow the child to demonstrate what he or she can do.

This work is in line with the response to intervention ideas first proposed in reading programmes. The first step is a universal programme in which all children will be involved; the partnership includes teachers, parents and therapists and aims at success for all pupils of all abilities. For children continuing to experience difficulties, differentiation takes place in the classroom and by observing their responses the partners can modify strategies and approaches for individual children. The school stays as the context, allowing partners access to a maximum amount of time and maximum numbers of pupils.

In the P4C model each child has an individual profile and a programme of work is derived directly from this profile. The children are taught both individually and in groups, where common objectives overlap. This is an example of how profiles can lead to the effective support a child should receive. The P4C process takes the information that is collected and progresses through a series stages to arrive at the best possible solution for that particular child. It is an individual programme, but not delivered individually. For best practice, it is probably better to deliver the programme in a group context in the course of daily life, such that the situation is ecologically valid, and the child is in an inclusive environment.

Participation is part of an ever-moving dynamic system. As the child's learning improves, the skills can be used in increasingly more complex ways, thereby increasing participation. Conversely, with increased participation through the affordance offered by the environmental context, the child has more opportunities to learn.

The recurring figure through this text is shown below (Fig. 5.4) but with slightly different headings. In this, optimum participation is obtained through modification of the environment in which the activity occurs, enhancing access through a variety of means. Once the child is in the learning situation the manner of presentation is optimized to the child's ability, thus increasing the time spent on a specific activity.

### Aggregation of marginal gains

Another related principle that is connected to both participation and learning is the **aggregation of marginal gains**. This concept has been around for a long time and is one that has strong face validity. In recent times it has increased in visibility by its use in the sporting world. The idea is that if performance of any skill can be improved by a small percentage in several different areas, the overall result has the potential to be large. This concept has been utilized widely in cycling where the minutia of every

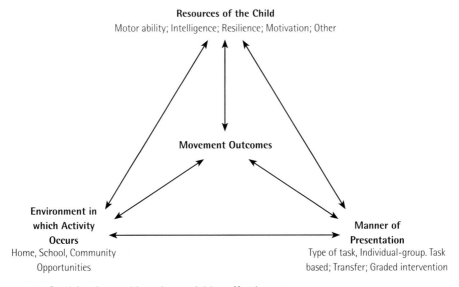

**Figure 5.4** Participation and learning variables affecting outcomes.

aspect of the rider, and support systems have been analysed and individually tailored. The programme includes detailed examination of all areas that will affect a sports person's performance, such as the individual's needs, daily routines, including hygiene, sleep and diet, achievable goals, equipment including clothing and cycles, training regimes and comfort in hotels. This information is shared with different professionals and most importantly the key individuals who coordinate the lifestyle regimen. It is the summation of these numerous small gains that have made the difference in overall performance. Although these actions would not, on their own, seem remarkable, the cumulative result is. One of the challenges is how marginal gains are coordinated into the aggregated whole. For a child with movement difficulties we can look for gains in small areas, such as effected by parents and family members, friends and colleagues, education, health and community systems and the individuals themselves. All these gains are tailored to the needs and resources of the individual.

The concept of small gains in a number of areas fits in with the concept of intervening in an ecological manner. Different individuals in a child's life bringing small changes that minimally alter aspects of the context and delivery. These can cause overall major changes in the way a child functions in daily activities. It is here that the named person/ movement coach (described in Chapter 4) would ensure that these small gains are easily built into the child's life so that they become routine and not an 'add-on'.

To achieve these small gains we can loosely delineate the roles of the various individuals in a child's life, who can contribute and to whom the named person/movement coach would look to involve. For example, the therapist can engage the child in formal practice on specific skills, such as handwriting, and this can be supplemented by more informal activities with the family, such as keeping a diary.

While occupational therapists and physiotherapists regularly work with children showing movement difficulties, they see the children so infrequently that it is not enough to evoke change. It has been likened, to going on a diet on Thursday afternoon only! But the message is clear: short regular sessions built into the fabric of daily life are more effective. Thus, the solution would be for the therapists to cascade their skills to the teachers so they can be utilized as continuously as possible in the course of the child's daily life at school.

A similar situation arises with parents and carers. They not only see the children for longer than anyone else, they also know the child better and have, of course, a huge vested interested in their well-being. A cascade model is also recommended for the parents and carers, with guidelines from health professionals and teachers to help them support their children. This type of support has the advantage of offering skilled help to those whose contact with children is greatest. It contains the best of all worlds with health professionals providing their specialist help in more formal sessions and teachers and parents modifying

> **Box 5.1** Ecology of participation and learning using marginal gain
>
> Participation and learning are bidirectional – a change in one changes the other.
> Participation involves changing the ecology of the setting to an inviting environment.
> Changing the ecological setting brings more child participation.
> More child participation brings better learning, if practices are appropriate.
> Small gains in many areas (accumulation of marginal gains) build up to a larger overall improvement.
> The small changes can be built into the daily life of the child such that they become routine.
> The named person/movement coach to work together to ensure that the life of the individual is subject to only minor changes that can easily be accommodated.

the daily life of the children in small but multiple ways to make a difference. In this way, the routines are modified only slightly, but because there are many of them, the overall effect will be great. This is the aggregation of marginal gains in ecological settings.

From the above, it may seem that there is the danger of the child being overloaded with sessions and intervention methods. To avoid this, the health professionals may want to do some specific practice sessions once a week or every two weeks, while the parents and teachers make small changes to the daily routines. All of this requires careful preparation, and it is here that the role of the **named person/movement coach** becomes important in ensuring careful planning and organization. The principles paramount here are the wishes of the child, within certain constraints, and the empowerment of parents. Practical examples of this are given in Chapter 4. Box 5.1 shows the relationship between the ecology of participation and learning using the concept of the accumulation of marginal gains.

## Developing objectives

*Multiple sources*
In order to develop objectives, the resources of the child are itemized in detail, the contextual opportunities for enhanced participation are identified and the support for the individual can be specified.

The next stage is to develop objectives with a robust plan; an objective without a robust plan is simply a wish! So how do we develop objectives that are suitable for the child? These can come from several sources including the parents, teachers, health professionals and, of course, the children themselves. However, not all these individuals will come to the same conclusion with respect to objectives. Teachers will obviously want to implement what they see as the most important objectives in an educational setting. Parents see what the child needs at home and health professionals will want to be guided by the reports from their various assessments. Any formal diagnosis would come about as a result of all of input from these individuals, with a qualified person making the final diagnosis. The child, however, may have different objectives. Indeed, work done by Dunford et al. (2005) showed that following assessment, teachers and parents were mainly in agreement about what the objectives should be. However, when the children were asked what they would like to do they gave much more specific answers such as 'I want to be able to ride my bicycle' or 'I would like to get dressed more quickly after a PE lesson'. If this is the case, then some form of compromise is needed, with the wishes of the children and the parents being paramount.

To make progress here, we need to look at the kind of support that can be given and combine this with the information each person contributes. For example, teachers see the children daily and they can effectively deliver a programme of support (Sugden and Chambers 2003). Thus, their view should be influential. Equally, parents and carers have the biggest vested interest other than the child. They can modify the child's daily life in small ways that will aggregate to make big changes and benefits in the child's life. Skilled movement professionals, such as occupational therapists and physiotherapists, have expert knowledge in this field and can engage with parents and teachers to reach an agreement. However, none of this can go ahead without the cooperation, motivation and participation of the child. For the child to be engaged one can either conduct a simple interview to find out their views or use an instrument, such as the Perceived Efficacy and Goal Setting (PEGS) (Missiuna et al. 2004), to find an agreed support through this method.

The PEGS instrument contains a set of 24 pictures organized in pairs with one showing a competent child and the other a child with difficulties. The children are asked to show which picture most resembles them and from this their choice of objectives can be derived. Dunford et al. (2005) used PEGS and found the children more likely to choose self-care and leisure activities as their objectives than teachers and parents. The children, obviously, want to play with their friends and not be embarrassed in delaying people when dressing and washing, and so on. Parents and teachers did not raise as many concerns in these areas. Studies such as this show that engaging children's views is important.

*Coming to agreement*
In most cases, it is relatively easy to come to agreement on the objectives and goals. When there is disagreement it is often with the child wanting slightly different objectives and goals. When this is the case then some compromising must be made. For example, if between the interested parties there are around six objectives, then, with the child's agreement individuals can take it in turns to specify theirs. Parents may say that the

| Box 5.2 Determining objectives | |
| --- | --- |
| **Who** | **How** |
| Home | Parent checklists interviews |
| School | Reports, teacher interviews, classroom observations |
| Health | Occupational therapists and physiotherapists and PTs, clinical reports and observations; paediatrican reports |
| Child | Interviews, questionnaires |

child can have three of theirs and the other three can be those of the professionals and parents. This is usually the case where more than one objective is specified. But how do we make the decision as to which objective to start with? Box 5.2 shows the variables to consider in order to determine specific objectives.

## Making priorities of objectives

A child with movement difficulties will most likely have several areas that require support, especially if they have co-occurring difficulties. These co-occurring difficulties can range from social ones, planning and organization, executive functioning problems or problems with attention, with or without hyperactivity. Thus, it is usual to have some criteria that can be used to determine priorities. Box 5.3 shows the criteria that have been used by various clinicians and researchers to determine priority. These are explained below.

*Child choice*
The child's choice has to be dealt with in a sensible manner. The child may choose objectives that are totally inappropriate; if so, some form of compromise needs to be reached by negotiation. The child may have difficulty in choosing and so again presentation of choices may help.

| Box 5.3 Criteria for prioritizing objectives |
| --- |
| ✓ Child choice |
| ✓ Most debilitating |
| ✓ Quick and easy wins |
| ✓ Enjoyment |
| ✓ Knock-on effect |
| ✓ Learning to move; moving to learn |

*Most debilitating*

If the child has a difficulty in their everyday life that is distressing and/or functionally restricting, then this is a strong reason for making this a priority objective. For example, in a young child, dressing and other self-care activities in a public place, such as after a physical education lesson at school, or even trying to dress early in the morning to go to school, can be good reasons to approach these tasks as a first step. In later childhood, it may be that the individual is poor at keyboard skills, thereby restricting social communication via mobile phones and other devices. Or, recreationally, the individual may become isolated by not being able to ride a bicycle with his friends. It may be that social difficulties are causing as much concern as the motor problems, but there is no reason why, with clever intervention, both cannot be addressed at the same time. All of these would be good reasons to choose them as a priority, with the proviso that context and how the individual responds should be taken into consideration.

*Quick and easy wins*

There are several ways to entice a child into activity and success is clearly one of them. Thus, if there is a task that is known that the child will enjoy and that they could achieve success in quite quickly, then this is a strong rational for using it. When using this method, ensure that the attribution theory of motivation is employed. In other words, if the child is successful let him or her know that it is because of their effort and ability and not just because the task was easy or they were lucky. If the individual has had restricted access to using a keyboard, then short, sharp practice sessions on a keyboard often bring good results. The individual can also practice these activities in private, which is often a good strategy for success.

*Enjoyment*

This aspect should not to be underestimated and carries with it a number of social and emotional effects. However, care must be exercised here as the child could use enjoyment as a comfort factor and not seek to progress. It is a good starting point, however, to gain the child's attention and increase motivation.

*Knock-on effects*

This criterion involves choosing objectives that are not only an end in themselves but, if successful, will lead to other gains. For example, in dealing with attention problems, motor activities that could enhance the overall attention of a child could be used. The use of movement to acquire other skills is the classic 'moving to learn' paradigm. In a similar vein, with older children we may concentrate on bicycle riding skills to promote and enhance their social activities. Cooperation games are also to be encouraged in order to foster better social skills, especially games and activities where success depends upon two or more children working together. Increasing

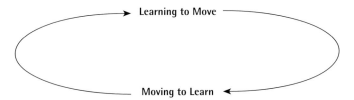

**Figure 5.5** Learning to move and moving to learn.

proficiency in handwriting may lead to higher marks and all round improvement in academic ability.

The criteria for developing priorities are not fixed and tend to involve subjective evaluations. For example, the child may be adamant about a particular a priority and this is very difficult to ignore. There may be some compromises to be made, but the motivation of the child, his or her satisfaction and the keenness to get on with learning are paramount.

*Learning to move; moving to learn*
As Figure 5.5 shows, outcomes from movement can be both the movement skills themselves and learning other skills through movement.

When **learning to move**, the child acquires those movement skills that are useful and often essential to their daily life. They will change according to age and ecological context, but at a young age, self-care skills are important as are the gross motor skills that allow them to join other children in their play activities. Fine motor skills such as handwriting and keyboards skills together with other manual skills are important. As the child develops, activities may change, for example to bicycle riding and later still, driving.

**Moving to learn** activities provide the opportunities for an individual to learn other skills through movement. Sharing, cooperation, patience, and teamwork are just a few of the skills that can be enhanced through appropriate movement activities. A child with attention difficulties can be helped by gradually increasing the attention demands of a motivating movement task. A child with social difficulties can be supported by movement activities that involve a partner.

In Chapter 2 we noted that the way in which tasks are taught or therapy is delivered is important. Crucial parts of this process involve providing instructions, explanations, demonstrations and feedback. We know that these actions are influenced by the age and ability of the child and the stage of learning reached. For example, for children with quite severe difficulties or those at an early stage of learning or are young, it is useful to give them no more than two points on which to concentrate. The points should be important and easy to understand. As the learning progresses, or with an older child, so does the complexity and detail of the information provided.

## Models of progression in learning

In this section we will look at the teaching and therapy contexts and how the stages influence the type of instructions and feedback that are given.

### Demonstrations, instructions and feedback

#### From understanding to automaticity

With children with difficulties or young children, we know that the early part of learning the task is getting to know what is required. Thus, the instructions should be short and minimal, but clear enough for the child to understand what to do in the first instance. Detailed feedback is not required here; it is sufficient to provide information so that the child 'gets the idea' of the task. Demonstrations are useful as long as they are accurate and easy to copy. For example, a simple right-handed throw with the contralateral left foot in front will suffice in the first instance. There is no need to say anything about body rotation or arm placement or lifting the foot for more leverage. As the learning progresses more detailed explanations and feedback can be given and a better technique can be encouraged, if necessary. In a task like this it is always useful to have some form of motivation, such as big target. As soon as the child can throw with some reasonable form and accuracy, the throw can be altered for distance and accuracy. More elaborate instructions can be given, with appropriate demonstrations and feedback as the child progresses.

As the child becomes more competent, the task can be altered to make it more challenging, such as throwing while moving, walking and then running. The child is now moving from understanding through consistency to adaptability. Providing instructions, explanations, demonstrations and feedback will vary according to where the child is in the learning process. (Fitts and Posner 1967; Gentile 2001). Box 5.4 illustrates how instructions and feedback change with skill progression.

> **Box 5.4** From understanding to automaticity of skill progression
>
> ✓ At first instructions are short and focus on the main point
> ✓ Any demonstration must link to the instructions
> ✓ Short feedback points given with progressions
> ✓ More detailed feedback given
> ✓ More challenging situations that require adaptation given
> ✓ Task is automatic and second task performed simultaneously

*Freezing to freeing degrees of freedom: a constraints dynamical systems approach*
A different way to look at the learning process is the dynamical systems approach first advocated by Bernstein (1967) and followed by Turvey (1977), Kelso (1995) and Thelen (1995). In this approach, learning progresses through a continuing attunement of the body to the environmental demands. In the early stages of learning, fewer degrees of freedom (DoF) (freezing; DoF) will be used for a given task progressing to more DOF (freeing DOF) being used as the child becomes more accomplished. This progression allows the child to adapt more efficiently to the changing environmental circumstances. In the parlance of the proponents, it involves a progression from the freezing to the freeing and exploiting the DoF. Instructions, demonstrations and feedback facilitate movement from rigid and fixed to flexible and adaptable. Box 5.5 illustrates the effect of this approach from simple biomechanical movements to those involving multiple and complex DoF.

Newell (1985) has, like others, proposed a three-level summary of motor learning, but from a constraints viewpoint, invoking many of the points from the dynamical systems model as shown in Box 5.5. His first stage involves the initial **assembling of a coordination pattern**. There are a large number to choose from and eventually the child picks one where the large number of DoF have been reduced. This will give a consistent response, but is lacking in adaptability. The next stage involves gaining control of a coordinative structure or collection of joints and muscles that are constrained to act as a single unit. This involves much exploration and searching and a reconfiguration of the motor system and DoF, such that the coordinative structures are more open to context. These are not in a fixed store but are flexible to meet the prevailing contextual conditions. In the third stage, there is the exploitation of the environmental information sources, with force, amplitude and direction all being considered in relation to optimal energy efficiency. This stage is often exemplified by top class sports people, such as a cover drive in cricket or jump shot in basketball. Box 5.6 shows the progression from consistent patterns to those that are more adaptable to the environmental context.

One can take any of these models and the same variables of instructions, demonstrations, explanations and feedback will apply. The concept of moving from simple delivery to

---

**Box 5.5** Freezing to freeing degrees of freedom

✓ Movements at first involving simple limb components (freezing DoF)
✓ Tasks organized for simple limb movements
✓ Tasks increased in complexity requiring adaptability
✓ Limbs becoming flexible and adapting to the demands of the task (freeing DoF)

> **Box 5.6** From assembling a coordination pattern to flexible exploitation of environmental information with differing forces, direction and amplitude
>
> ✓ Choosing a consistent coordination pattern but that is not adaptable
> ✓ Gaining control of coordination, such as limbs, joints acting as a single unit – a coordinative structure
> ✓ Exploitation of environmental context to optimize adaptability and energy efficiency

a more complex one remains the same. In all the above models, instructions, explanations, demonstrations and feedback will change according to what part of the learning process the child is engaged in. In our practical examples in Chapter 7 we will show how these would change, according to the profile of the child.

## Case studies

In Chapter 4 we detailed six case studies, three from DCD and three from other developmental disorders. Here we look at each one again to illustrate how objectives and priorities for action may be developed from the profiles. Below are summaries of the detail on each case presented in Chapter 4.

### Case studies of developmental coordination disorder

#### A review of Adam

Adam is a 7-year-old boy of average ability in his schoolwork but who has struggled with his motor skills since he was a toddler. His parents noticed his delays but were not overly concerned until he went to school and the delay seemed to be holding him back in some of the classroom activities involving manual activities. In physical education classes his teacher reported that he was 'clumsy' and 'awkward' compared to other children. He is good-natured but now starting to receive some teasing as he cannot ride a bicycle; he is a slow writer and has problems with planning and organization. The MABC-2 Checklist (Henderson et al. 2007) was completed on him by his teacher and parents and he had an overall score that placed him in the 8th to 10th centile on Sections A and B. In section C he was scored as hesitant, forgetful and disorganized, but good on the rest of the items; however, he was starting to be upset by failure. On the MABC-2 Test Adam scored at the 2nd centile, with difficulties in manual dexterity and balance. Thus, on the MABC-2 Test and Checklist he would fulfill Criteria A and B from DSM-5 (APA 2013). He was examined by a paediatrician who noted no neurological abnormalities and the school reported no real delay in his academic achievement. In diagnostic terms he could be given a diagnosis of DCD. Box 5.7 summarizes Adam's profile.

**Box 5.7** Summary of Adam's profile

**Objectives and priorities**

From discussions with Adam, his parents, teacher and therapist, the following objectives and priorities were developed:

✓ Speedier handwriting – all agreed this was a priority. The MABC-2 also identified poor manual skills as a concern. An improvement in this area would not only improve his handwriting but also hopefully facilitate other tasks in school requiring manual skills. As an example, Figure 5.6 shows a young boy practicing his writing.

✓ Bicycle riding – only Adam placed an emphasis on this as he thought it would help him to be able to play with his peers.

These two items were the ones that were identified to work on first. All agreed on the first one, but only Adam on the second. His parents, teachers and therapist thought bicycle riding would be a challenge for him, but Adam was clear that he wanted to do this and it was, therefore, accepted.

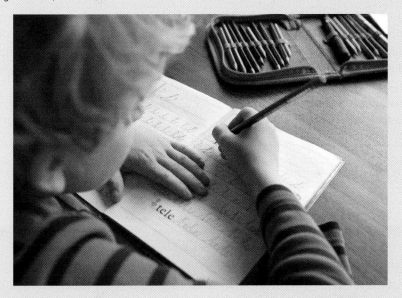

**Figure 5.6** Young boy writing.

The two objectives were established as the ones on which to work. He had other difficulties that were identified, such as planning and organization and hesitancy and forgetfulness. But although they were noted by his teacher and parents, it was decided to try to encourage these on an informal basis during directed support and intervention. Adam is a good-natured boy within a normal range of ability and it is thought these characteristics, together with a supportive environment, would aid the accomplishment of the two priority objectives. They might have some spin-off effects on his planning and organizational skills.

*A review of Jenny*

Jenny is a 13-year-old girl, highly intelligent, quiet and reserved who has had a history of neuromata difficulties; she was delayed in rolling, sitting, standing, and walking. In her first year of life she was assessed for suspected cerebral palsy because she presented hypertonicity in her arms but this seemed to disappear and no diagnosis of cerebral palsy was ever given. She has had speech therapy over the years, but she still has an articulation difficulty, which she now finds embarrassing. She is an extremely high achiever at school, working on A-level mathematics at the age of 13. Her academic excellence is seen across the curriculum, except in areas where controlled movements are required, such as in physical education and laboratory activities. She is a very slow writer and does not text in public. Jenny is beginning to have difficulties socializing, although she has two close friends who support her, but she does not readily mix with her peer group in social activities, such as cycling or dancing. She is articulate and honest and would like help.

Both the MABC-2 Checklist and Test were administered to Jenny and, as expected, she scored in the lowest 1% in both. There were, however, some notable scores. On the Checklist she only scored a 'Yes' to underestimating her ability, being timid and becoming anxious; in all other behaviours she scored 'No'. This will be an advantage when it comes to building a profile. Jenny is very keen to try to improve, is clear in her profile and objectives and is looking for guidance as to how to achieve these. Box 5.8 summarizes Jenny's profile.

*Review of James*

James is 20 years of age and in his first year at university, studying chemistry. James has a history of movement difficulties and had a diagnosis of DCD at 9 years of age.

---

**Box 5.8** Summary of Jenny's profile

**Objectives and priorities**

From discussions with Jenny, her parents, teachers and therapist the following objectives and priorities were developed:

- ✓ Work on fine motor skills such as writing and texting. All agreed on this and thought a good way forward would be to involve her two close friends. These seem to be essential components of any intervention in this phase of Jenny's life.
- ✓ Communication, in terms of articulation and general socializing. Continuing with speech therapy but asking the therapist to cascade practices to Jenny's parents, teachers and others, so that they can be used in everyday life. Use of her two close friends to help her extend friendships.
- ✓ Use of 'easy' motor activities to help Jenny gain confidence and encourage more participation in motor activities. Success in these, with the help of her two close friends, will enable her to become less timid and maybe attempt slightly more difficult tasks in a supportive environment.

<br>

**Box 5.9** Summary of James' profile

**Objectives and priorities**

Following discussions with James and advice from the University Diversity Officer the following objectives and priorities were developed:

✓ Riding a bicycle is the first thing that James mentioned and said that if this could be accomplished it would change his life substantially. He does run but he maintained that it is not as social as cycling and so this is his first priority. This will take some care and attention as James has most difficulties when moving in a moving environment. Finding a bicycle-riding course for James may be problematic but will be explored and it may be that some tailored programme, supported by friends could be the way forward.

✓ Joining recreational clubs at university may be a way for James to interact socially with others. These need to be chosen with care, but could include various fitness classes that involve coordination activities, which would help with his coordination and with making friends.

Currently, it was not thought that learning to drive was a priority for two reasons: first, at university, a car is not a necessity and second, learning how to ride a bicycle may help with abilities such as moving in a changing environment, which will be necessary when he does start to learn to drive.

<br>

James' MABC-2 Test and Checklist scores from both parents and teachers showed quite severe difficulties in the areas of aiming and catching, balance, adjusting appropriately when the environment was moving or unpredictable. He also had difficulties in nearly all items of self-care and classroom skills, ball skills and recreational and physical education skills. On both the Test and the Checklist he was in the typical range on practically all areas of fine motor demands. Overall, he was between the 5th and 15th centile, which would be in the monitoring rather than immediate action range. However, his occupational therapist thought that his skills in the moving environment, balance and recreational skills were poor enough for her to recommend that Criteria A and B of DSM-IV were satisfied. On an IQ test he scored 136 with little discrepancy between verbal and performance scores. James was distressed about his poor motor skills, even though and ran in the school cross-country team. He enjoyed this activity as it kept him fit and healthy and gave him a social context. But he could not ride a bicycle and had not learned to drive, two activities he felt restricted his social life. He would like some guidance and support and being at university may help this. Box 5.9 summarizes James profile.

## Case studies of children with other developmental disorders

In Chapter 1 we described how children with movement difficulties could be placed broadly into two categories: those with movement difficulties as a primary defining condition such as the three we have described above and those who have another primary defining condition but also have movement difficulties as a secondary characteristic. The following children fit into this area.

*A review of Marie*

Marie is a 12-year-old girl just starting the first year at secondary school who has been diagnosed with attention-deficit disorder (ADD), primarily because of her attention difficulties not hyperactivity. Marie has daydreaming problems and has difficulty coming to attention. The diagnosis of ADD was given according to the DSM-IV criteria, as she evidenced more than six of the characteristics listed in diagnostic criteria A1. Her parents and her teachers were given the Connors Checklist to complete and, again, the low attention scores were noted. In class she scored around the 25th centile in most subjects but had no extra support. As she grew up, problems started to become more apparent at home. Her gross motor skills have been poor throughout her childhood, mainly because she rarely participated in any physical activity in or out of school. She cannot ride a bicycle and her fine motor skills were also poor. She was slow to dress in the mornings being distracted and often missed school buses. She has low self-concept and it is difficult to disentangle her poor motor skills from her ADD and other social and emotional characteristics. She has low self-esteem, which is not helped by her poor motor performance. All agree that she needs to participate more, and that movement can act both as an end it itself and as an aid to overcoming some of her attention difficulties. Box 5.10 summarizes Marie's profile.

---

**Box 5.10** Summary of Marie's profile

**Objectives and priorities**

After discussions with Marie, her parents and teachers the following objectives and priorities were agreed:

✓ All feel that encouraging and facilitating participation in movement situations will help both her motor skills and her attention. To facilitate participation, the context/environment will need to be more accommodating to her needs.

✓ Provide motor activities that are quickly achievable, but need some attention to achieve success. This will not only aid her attention but also build her confidence and increase her self-esteem. These motor activities in the ideal scenario should involve her two close friends who have empathy with her difficulties and are willing to help. Marie may choose which tasks she would like to learn, such as dressing quickly, texting or any skill that she feels she really needs. Figure 5.7 shows a girl like Marie practicing her texting.

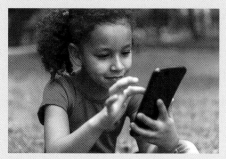

**Figure 5.7** A girl like Marie practicing her texting.

*Review of Andrew*

Andrew is a 9-year-old boy who was diagnosed with high functioning autism. (Asperger syndrome under the DSM-IV criteria) at age 5. This has led to him being disadvantaged socially and at school. At 2 to 3 years of age he had lack of appropriate use of language and other forms of communication such as eye contact and hugging and touching. At 4 to 5 years of age his speech was syntactically good but the context in which it was used was highly inappropriate language was usually one sided. Along with Asperger syndrome, Andrew has motor difficulties that unfortunately are now becoming a source of stress for him. His classmates are now less tolerant of his behaviours. He is clumsy, cannot ride a bicycle and has a bizarre running style. This is causing him distress and making him more isolated in and outside of school, where he has few friends.

When Andrew discusses his difficulties he does it solely from his viewpoint but does recognize that others may be able to help him. His parents and teachers feel a new approach is required as he enters the last years of primary school to help him cope in secondary school. Box 5.11 summarizes Andrew's profile.

*Review of Paul*

Paul is a 14-year-old boy in a mainstream secondary school. He has no specified diagnosis for any condition, but he underachieves in several areas with knock-on effects to his self-esteem, self-concept and few friendships in and out of school. From an early age, Paul was delayed in his motor skills, language and other forms of communication and generally did not seem as inquisitive as his siblings had been. He does not show

---

**Box 5.11** Summary of Andrew's profile

**Objectives and priorities**

After discussions with Andrew, his parents and teachers, the following objectives and priorities were developed and agreed:

✓ All were agreed that making friends should be the main objective and that all other objectives could feed into this. There is strong evidence that individuals with ASD cope much better if they have a few supportive friends who understand them and have empathy. In addition, teachers and parents thought that this objective could lead to the successful accomplishment of other objectives, such as communication skills. Movement situations that involve cooperation will encourage communication with others and, hopefully, help him to develop friendships.

✓ For Andrew, learning to ride a bicycle was his highest priority and the most important to him. His teachers and parents did not mention this as an objective but Andrew was adamant about it.

With Andrew, as with other individuals, movement activities are not only objectives in their own right, but also can aid to other accomplishments.

---

> **Box 5.12** Summary of Paul's profile
>
> **Objectives and priorities**
>
> After discussion with Paul, his parents and his teachers, the following objectives and priorities were agreed:
>
> ✓ Paul was very keen to develop his ball skills ability and so a programme of learning tennis is to be put into operation. Paul thought this was a good idea because it would involve interaction with others he knew and whom he believed would help him. His good social skills will be a real advantage here.
>
> ✓ He can ride a bicycle but he is not very confident and so he will be enrolled in a bicycle-riding scheme. He believes this will help his friendships.

typical peer interaction. He was slow in learning to read and is now at a level two years below his chronological age expectation. His mathematics is at a similar level.

His motor skills are and always have been poor and he has had no support for these. He was delayed in walking and this continued with most of his fundamental motor skills, both gross and fine.

Paul is keen to learn most things, but is now starting to worry he will either fail or be shown to take much longer to learn than his friends. He has been tested in a number of areas and found to be, on average, between the 15th and 20th centiles. This is a common profile, with no formal diagnosis, but enough symptoms to give parents, teachers and Paul some concern. He is aware of the difficulties and he is now at a stage where he is watching other children progress in most areas and which is causing his level of self-concept and self-esteem to fall. Working on his motor skills can play a role here, but only as part of an overall approach addressing his other difficulties. Box 5.12 summarizes Paul's profile.

## Summary

This chapter has sought to bridge the gap between the collection of information about an individual child and the actual practical work with children. This is outlined more in Chapters 6 and 7. Several working principles have been identified that apply to all children. The first is that the set of resources a child possesses and brings to the movement situation is the starting point from which all else flows. This is the same for all children. They all live in a social context with the constraints of the wider environment and the way in which support is given affects their participation and learning. Small changes in a number of these areas will alter the manner of participation and learning and, thus, the competence of the child. The information and subsequent agreement about the objectives of any programme come from multiple sources. Therefore, compromises often have to be made to ensure, as far as possible, that all interested parties are comfortable with the programme. The priority given to these objectives have multiple influences, but the overriding one will be the views of the child.

We know that for a child to learn, the environment must be inviting enough for him or her to want to participate. This occurs at various levels. At a macro level, the wider social context of the child's world needs to accommodate the individual child's needs. The home, community and school will play major roles in this, often having to accommodate change. Once the child is participating more, learning can progress and the way in which instructions and demonstrations and feedback are given will all play a major part.

# References

APA (2002) *Diagnostic and Statistical Manual of Mental Disorder*, 4th edition. (DSM-IV) Arlington, VA: American Psychiatric Association.

Bernstein N (1967) *The Coordination and Regulation of Movements*. New York: Pergamon Press.

Blank R, Barnett AL, Cairney J, et al. (2019) International clinical practice recommendations on the definition, diagnosis, assessment, intervention, and psychosocial aspects of developmental coordination disorder. *Dev Med Child Neurol* 61: 242–285.

Cairney J, Hay JA, Veldhuizen S, Missiuna CL, Fraught BE (2010) Developmental coordination disorder, sex, and activity deficit over time: a longitudinal analysis of participation trajectories in children with and without coordination difficulties. *Dev Med Child Neurol* 52: 67–72.

Chambers ME, Sugden DA (2014) Intervention for young children displaying coordination disorders. *J Early Childhood Res* 14: 115–131.

Conners CK, Sitarenios G, Parker JDA, Epstein JN (1998) The Revised Conners' Parent Rating Scale (CPRS-R): Factor Structure, Reliability, and Criterion Validity. *J Abnorm Child Psychol* 26: 257–268.

Dunford C, Missiuna C, Street E, Sibert J (2005) Children's perceptions of the impact of developmental coordination disorder on activities of daily living. *Br J Occup Ther* 68: 207–214.

Engel-Yeger B, Kasis AH (2010) The relationship between developmental co-ordination disorders, child's perceived self-efficacy and preference to participate in daily activities. *Child Care, Health Dev* 36: 670–677.

Fitts PM, Posner MI (1967) *Human Performance*. Oxford, UK: Brooks/Cole.

Gentile AM (2000) Skill acquisition: action movement and neuromotor processes. In Carr J, Shepard RB (eds). *Movement Science: Foundations for Physical Therapy in Rehabilitation*, 2nd edition. Gaithersburg, MD: Aspen.

Henderson SE, Sugden DA, Barnett AE (2007) *Movement Assessment Battery for Children*, 2nd edition. Pearson: London.

Kelso JAS (1995) *Dynamic Patterns: The Self-organization of Brain and Behavior*. Cambridge, MA: MIT Press.

Magalhães LC, Cardoso AA, Missiuna C (2011) Activities and participation in children with developmental coordination disorder: a systematic review. *Res Dev Disabil* 4: 1309–1316.

Missiuna C, Pollack N, Law M (2004) *Perceived Efficacy of Goal Setting in Young Children (PEGS).* San Antonio, TX: Psychological Corporation.

Missiuna C, Pollock N, Campbell W, et al. (2017) Using an innovative model of service delivery to identify children who are struggling in school. *Br J Occup Ther* 80: 145–154.

Missiuna C, Pollack MA, Levac DE, Russell D (2012) Partnering for change: An innovative school based occupational therapy service delivery model for children with developmental coordination disorder. *Can J Occup Ther* 79: 141–150.

Newel KM (1985) Coordination, control and skill. *Adv Psychol* 27: 295–317.

Sugden DA, Chambers ME (2003) Intervention in children with DCD: the role of parents and teachers. *Br J Educ Psychol* 73: 545–561.

Sugden DA, Chambers ME (eds) (2006) *Children with Developmental Coordination Disorder.* London: Whurr.

Sugden DA, Chambers ME (2007) Stability and change in children with developmental coordination disorder. *Child Health Care Dev* 33: 520–528.

Sugden DA, Henderson SE (2007) *Ecological Intervention for Children with Movement Difficulties.* Pearson: London.

Thelen E (1995) Motor development: a new synthesis. *Am Psychol* 50: 79–95.

Turvey MT (1977) Preliminaries to a theory of action with reference to vision. In Shaw R, Bransford J (eds). *Perceiving, Acting and Knowing.* Hillsdale NJ: Erlbaum, pp. 211–265.

World Health Organization (2001) *International Classification of Functioning, Disability and Health (ICF).* Geneva: World Health Organization.

# Chapter 6
## Specific intervention guideline

### Learning motor skills

In the preceding chapters, we have detailed general principles underlying both assessment and intervention together with examples of case studies. In this chapter we will outline how we can enact a support and intervention programme. Specific details will be given in the Case Studies in Chapter 7.

How an individual learns motor skills has been the topic of investigations for over a century, in contexts ranging from the workplace, sporting arenas and rehabilitation (Revie and Larkin 1993; Mandich et al. 2001; Davids et al. 2008; Schmidt and Lee 2011). Classic texts such as Schmidt and Lee (2011) have provided great detail on the motor learning process. All of these have provided insights into the optimum conditions to facilitate this acquisition process in order to set up the best learning environment for individuals with movement difficulties. In Chapter 2 we noted that learning is a process containing a contextually based problem. All of this is encapsulated with our core figure repeated below (Figure 6.1) from most of our chapters, that learning outcomes are a function of the dynamic relationship between the resources of the child, the type of task and manner of presentation and the context in which learning takes place both in the narrow and wider sense. Learning never involves simply the child as the unit of analysis; it is the child in both narrow and wider contexts. This chapter mainly concentrates on the bottom right hand corner of Figure 6.1, the Manner of Presentation.

This figure represents the three areas to work on. The child resources are the obvious desired outcomes from any intervention. In this section, we will look at how everyday

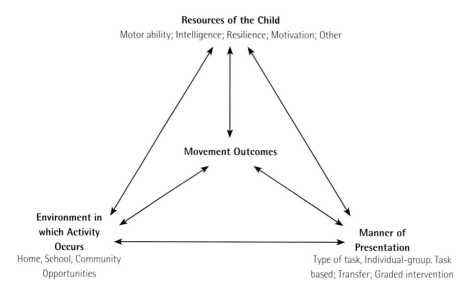

**Figure 6.1** The Manner of Presentation.

skills are taught and how the principles of learning can best optimize this process. However, we should not forget the context in which these skills are taught, as depicted in the bottom left-hand corner of the Figure. One can utilize various models of ecological theory to describe these models but all should involve parents, teachers, and professionals working together to provide the optimal learning environment. A good example of these, described already on page 104, is the Partnering for Change model (Missiuna et al. 2011).

## Evidence for our guidelines

Whenever intervention and support is being discussed or evaluated there are a number of decisions that have to be made: What type of intervention should be used? How long it should last? Who should deliver it? Who makes the choices and how it is taught? In the following sections, we examine a number of the decisions that have to be made before implementing support and intervention practices.

### Theoretical, empirical and professional evidence

There are a number of sources of evidence that can provide guidelines for these decisions. In Chapter 4 we noted that evidence come in three forms: **theoretical, empirical and professional** (Sugden and Dunford 2007). Most research has been carried out on empirical support through randomized controlled trials, systematic reviews and meta-analyses. But we know these are not the total answer. First, because while evidence is abundant, it can be limited by the different inclusion criteria of the studies included in the meta-reviews. Second, without a sound base, any evidence is incomplete. We have a number of competing and converging bases for our work and we include summaries of the major ones. Third, professional input is always worthy of inclusion as it taps into the skills and knowledge of clinicians and other individuals who are working directly with children and young adults. Later in this chapter we will present our guidelines using these three sources of evidence.

Intervention is about the variables of how individuals learn. Chapter 2 outlined some examples of what the results of learning would show. These involved new skills, improvement and adaptability. Basut we would also include more qualitative outcomes such as smoothness of the movement, how effortless the movement looks and how the top performer achieves this quality of movement, often with minimal effort.

Our evidence-base for intervention guidelines is growing and with the recent publication of the International Clinical Practice guidelines (Blank et al. 2019), these guidelines are now more secure. The evidence for intervention in children with movement difficulties is almost as abundant as for other bodies of literature, on attention-deficit–hyperactivity disorder, autism spectrum disorder and other developmental disorders, as well as sport. This is particularly true when we examine such variables as practice sessions: how they are structured, for how long, and how to provide instructions and feedback. In this chapter, we aim to translate the evidence for intervention it into the teaching and therapy sessions.

Much of the time when we talk of intervention we use the word 'teaching'. We do this because both parents and teachers are more familiar with this word than say 'therapy'. However, we also recognize that specialist advice and support is given by therapists who use the word 'therapy'. We do not discuss the semantic difference between the two words, but emphasize that we use teaching to include both, and both are aimed at supporting, facilitating and guiding children through the learning process.

## Systematic reviews and meta-analyses

Much of our evidence for support for intervention methods comes from empirical work in the form of systematic reviews or meta-analyses. A **systematic review** involves answering a research question by collecting and summarizing the empirical evidence on the topic using pre-specified eligibility criteria. Thus, the results of a number of studies that meet the criteria are examined and summarized in a qualitative manner. A **meta-analysis** employs statistical methods to summarize the results of systematic reviews but uses more specialist, statistical terms to describe the results. A third type of evidence are **meta-reviews** that collate the results of meta-analyses and systematic reviews.

Over the last 20 years a number of articles, reviews and meta-anlayses have addressed the efficacy of intervention methods for children with movement disorders, especially in individuals with DCD (Simms et al. 1996; Mandich et al. 2001; Polatajko et al. 2001a and b; Larkin and Parker 2002; Wilson 2005; Hillier 2007; Sugden 2007; Roley 2009; Camden et al. 2014). While this is not an exhaustive list it does illustrate that intervention has been taken seriously since before the turn of the century.

In this section, we present the results of three recent systematic reviews, meta-analyses and meta-reviews, followed by a scoping review. From these and those listed above we generate general guidelines and then articulate them with theoretical and professional issues in order to present our recommendations. We stress that these are not the only form of evidence that we will use but they will guide our thinking and intervention planning.

*Example 1  A meta-analysis*
A meta-analysis by Smits-Engelsman et al. (2013) used a variety of databases between 1995 and 2011 to examine outcome interventions using a number of descriptive terms such as DCD, dyspraxia, motor difficulties, and perceptual motor difficulties. It examined a range of intervention methods including physiotherapy, occupational therapy sensory integration, cognitive orientation to daily occupational performance (CO-OP), neuromotor task training (NTT), perceptual motor training, task specific training, and kinaesthesis training. All these were assessed by two independent experts using the PEDro scales.

This was a comprehensive search, looking at the level of evidence, including effect sizes, from over 3700 papers. They eventually identified 26 articles that met the full criteria for a meta-analysis. Several tests were used in the study for assessment with the MABC being favoured. (MABC-2 Henderson, Sugden and Barnett (2007)).

The conclusions were similar to the ones recommended by the Leeds Consensus Statement (Sugden 2006), see Box 6.1. These were task specific functional approaches, relevant to

---

**Box 6.1** Results from Smits-Engelsman et al. review (2013)

**The following interventions were recommended:**

✓ Task oriented approaches
✓ Traditional therapy
✓ One study on motor imagery

**Interventions not recommended were:**

✓ Process oriented approaches
✓ Those involving medication, such as methylphenidate

---

daily living and child centred, involving significant others such as parents and teachers and grounded in sound theoretical concepts.

*Example 2 A systematic review*

A recent systematic review by Preston et al. (2016) looked at interventions for children with DCD. They used strict criteria for inclusion in the study (PRISMA; Moher et al. 2009). Systematic literature searches of six electronic databases were employed and a hand search of recent reviews and articles was also carried out.

The authors searched the literature from 2000 to 2016, identifying 846 articles, nine randomized, controlled trials and 15 intervention studies. Each article was studied by two independent reviewers and after a strict selection process, nine randomized controlled trials were identified.

The resulting focus centred on three types of studies: sports skills, task oriented and process oriented study.

The studies were divided into favourable or unfavourable outcomes, with either high or moderate confidence in each leading to strong or weak recommendations (see Box 6.2).

A major difference in the Preston et al. study compared to other studies, is that it excluded any randomized controlled trials investigating the CO-OP (Polataijko et al. 2001). They said this was because, the trials were not methodologically robust enough to include, despite the COOP being a commonly assessed and popular approach. From our evidence that includes theory, empiricism and professional practice reports, we would argue that the CO-OP is sufficiently robust and has strong supporting evidence from professionals in the field. We recognize however that the empirical criteria employed in the Peston et al. study argued against its inclusion but we would include it.

---

**Box 6.2** Results from the Preston et al. review (2016)

**Three approaches showed good evidence:**
- ✓ Task oriented motor training
- ✓ Neuromotor task training
- ✓ Motor imagery plus task training, although only a few studies were used for evaluation
- ✓ Perceptual motor training carried out by therapists

**Approaches that did not receive support**
- ✓ Process approaches looking at such areas as core stability
- ✓ A small number involving soccer training, WiiFit, aqua-therapy, table tennis and self-concept training

*Example 3  A meta-review*

A study by Miyahara et al. (2016) differs from the others in that it is a narrative meta-review that examined intervention outcomes for children with DCD. A search of electronic databases was conducted by two independent assessors. The AMSTAR system for review appraisal (Shea et al. 2007) was used, with scores of 0–3 indicating low; 4–7 medium and 8–11 high. This yielded 90 articles but only four met the criteria set by the authors. This article noted that many of the reviews they examined had numerous shortcomings and therefore concrete evidence for DCD interventions is not yet clearly defined.

*Example 4  A scoping review*

A different approach was taken by Camden et al. (2014) who employed a scoping review examining 500 documents using six databases and combining techniques on scholarly and grey literature. Thirty-one articles met their inclusion criteria with the recommendations, shown in Box 6.3.

When examining these studies and others, it is pertinent to remember that the type and number of drivers that are entered for the inclusion criteria to be included govern the results. One can see the difference between the Miyahara et al. review (2016) that included only four articles and the Smits-Engelsman et al. (2013) review that included 26 articles. Nevertheless, some common conclusions can be arrived at from the three recent reviews and analyses, together with studies preceding these three.

There are some anomalies, but in general there is more agreement than disagreement. It is clear from the majority of studies that intervention of any kind is better than none at all. Second, in the majority of studies there is consensus that task-oriented approaches using functional activities are preferable.

The scoping review of Camden et al. (2014) describes the bigger picture, using qualitative and quantitative data from a variety of sources. These together with the meta-analyses and reviews help us in planning support and intervention.

---

**Box 6.3** Results from Camden et al. (2014) scoping review

✓ Services to be organized to efficiently meet the comprehensive needs of children with DCD and their families.

✓ Orderly, defined pathways to ensure access to diagnosis, evaluation and intervention.

✓ A graduated, staged approach to foster capacity building to address the children's' and families' needs.

✓ Collaborative working between interested parties.

✓ Evidence-based intervention and services integrating child and family views.

✓ Fostering of function and participation, and prevention of sensory consequences.

We have taken the common agreements and merged them with our own ideas and practices, noting any differences or elaborations. The first point of debate focuses on what should be taught or provided in therapy. For this we look at the difference between what has been labelled **process approaches** versus **specific task approaches**. All of the papers and articles directly addressed DCD. In one respect, this is reasonable as DCD is the most commonly diagnosed motor difficulty in children. However, there are other children with developmental disorders who exhibit movement disorders and we have little information on them with regard to intervention for movement skills. Therefore, our recommendations will be taken from the general conclusions from the systematic reviews and meta-analyses, plus the scoping review. We will use them to present our guidelines, together with theoretical, empirical and professional information from the motor learning and development literature and from clinicians.

## What should we teach and how should we teach it?

In all interventions and support there are two underlying goals, either specifically stated or implied: first, that any skill is taught and retained over a reasonable period of time; second, that this skill can be modified and generalized so that it can be transferred to different contexts.

In order to achieve these two goals, support and intervention can be viewed at a macro or micro level. Therefore, one can start with the recommendations of Camden et al. (2014), following such innovations as the Partnering For Change model (see page 104; Missiuna et al. 2011) ideas and gradually moving to how individuals and specific skills are taught and transferred.

In the last 20 years there has been much discussion about the type of intervention that should be pursued with children showing movement disorders. Much of this has centred on children who are diagnosed with DCD as this is the most prevalent movement disorder among children. In this section, we analyse the different approaches and how the various proponents have classified them, together with the information that supports the different viewpoints. Various categories of intervention approaches have been identified, ranging from popular ones to others that are more idiosyncratic and rare.

The approaches can be divided into the two large categories: **task oriented approaches** and **process-oriented approaches**. Although this is a rather reductionist approach, these are the two most commonly used approaches when examining the effectiveness of intervention (Pless and Carlsson 2000; Schoemaker et al. 2003; Wilson 2005; Polatajko et al. 2006; Sugden 2007; Hillier 2011; Smits-Engelsman et al. 2013, 2015, 2016; Preston et al. 2016; Blank et al. 2019).

However, these categories are not as discrete as they are often portrayed. A simplistic view says that task approaches are simply that: one teaches the task that needs to be learned, such as riding a bicycle or forming letters. Similarly, process approaches aim to reinforce underlying processes, such as visual perception, kinaesthesis or core stability. The aim is to improve these processes so that they can be transferred to activities of every day living. These processes are not discrete; they form a continuum and one often contains the characteristics of another, Many of the intervention schemes involve some underlying processes. For example, the cognitive motor approach (Henderson and Sugden 1992), ecological intervention (Sugden and Henderson 2007) and the CO-OP (Polataijko et al. 2001), are all task approaches and include processes that involve cognition and perception. All would purport to be task-based but also involve some cognitive and/or sensory processes. Thus, one can teach a task that is an activity of everyday living, yet involve such cognitive processes as self-goal selection and setting, self-monitoring and problem solving.

Similarly, in process oriented approaches such as sensory Integration therapy, although the emphasis is on *processes*, particularly sensory ones, tasks are used in the intervention schedules. Sensory Integration therapy, now includes more task-oriented approaches and in many ways has changed from the original approach developed by Jean Ayres in the early 1970s.

The difference between the two approaches is the **primary objectives** of the programme. In task-based approaches the object is to teach tasks that are the end product. In the process approach the aim is to reinforce the underlying processes that the proponents purport to be common to a variety of tasks. However, one can argue that they are using different methods to achieve the same result: a generalization of what has been learned across a variety of tasks. One approach does it rather specifically and the other more indirectly. With this in mind we examine the differences and pros and cons of each approach.

*Task approaches*
At first glance, task approaches are relatively straightforward. Following assessment and the setting of objectives and priorities, the focus is on the task to be taught, for example, handwriting or ball skills. The task oriented approaches that have appeared to be the most successful are those that use cognitive methods and strategies to teach task-based functional skills. The task approaches are the ones that are most favoured by the Clinical Practice Guidelines (Blank et al. 2019).

This type of approach has good face validity. If the child has a particular problem in a specific area, then that area is directly addressed. There is a huge advantage and positivity about this approach, but it is not without its difficulties. For example, a child with multiple needs may have a number of tasks that require support, but there is insufficient time to address all these tasks.

An individual does not need to learn every single variation of a given skill in order to be competent. The answer then becomes one of transfer or generalization of the learned skills to different tasks.

How does one teach a skill or groups of skills so that they can be used in more than one situation, according to the contextual demand? It can be achieved through modification of the task and the environment and adjustments by the individual.

In the last two decades numerous review articles have that recommend task-oriented approaches (Revie and Larkin 1993; Polatajko et al. 1995; Pless and Carlsson 2000; Schoemaker et al. 2003; Wilson 2005; Sugden 2007; Blank et al. 2012; 2019).

*Process-oriented approaches*
Process-oriented approaches involve a number of loosely connected methods, many of them drawing on the work of Jean Ayres (Ayres 1979). They may differ in certain aspects but have common principles that involve the remediation of an underlying process or structure. This can be sensory, such as vision or kinaesthesis, or others involving more fundamental biological structures that improve the function of the cerebellum (Fawcett and Nicholson 1995; Nicholson and Fawcett 1999). They are usually based on the assumption that there is an underlying process that is deficient. They are 'bottom up' approaches that address the underlying processes of a skill and not the skill itself. The idea behind these approaches (see Box 6.4) is that if the underlying processes are

---

**Box 6.4** Task and process approaches

**Task approaches**
- ✓ Teaching or therapy for the actual task that is required
- ✓ Functional skills
- ✓ Use of cognitive strategies
- ✓ Good face validity
- ✓ Use of variability of practice
- ✓ Question about number of tasks to address and time available
- ✓ Strong supporting evidence from theory, empiricism and professional practice

**Process approaches**
- ✓ Remediation of underlying process or structure
- ✓ 'Bottom up' approaches attempting to address sensory mechanisms or biological substrates
- ✓ Generalization intended to be an advantage and goal
- ✓ Supporting theoretical and empirical evidence is lacking
- ✓ Supported by professionals

remediated then generalization can occur across a variety of surface skills and tasks. If a sensory process or the neural mechanism is improved, then improvement may be seen across tasks that include these components. While there is some evidence for the efficacy of this approach (Ayres 1979; Simms et al. 1996) robust evidence is not plentiful. A review by Roley and Jacobs (2009) suggests that there is a lack of studies with stringent research protocols. Other authors, such as Wilson (2005) note that the theoretical foundations of this approach are not based on modern theories of motor control and that the empirical evidence is at best inconclusive. Sugden and Wade (2013) conclude that more theoretical, empirical and professional evidence is required to justify the use of this approach. Certainly, the theoretical bases of process approaches often lie in outdated information processing models. However, these approaches have a large professional following, are taught widely in occupational therapy training courses and are supported by many professionals. They are mixed and matched with tasks, which moves them away from the original theoretical base.

## What can we learn from the motor learning literature?

In Chapter 2 we outlined a number of principles of motor learning. These have come from such diverse fields as rehabilitation following neural problems or injuries; the learning of skills in sports; the work place, such as cigar rolling; and the teaching of keyboard skills. Although there is not much of evidence on these topics with regard to children with movement difficulties, we believe the generic guidelines from motor learning can provide us with the tools on how to teach these children the skills they need in their daily lives. The following general points are those found to be successful over a wide range of fields and activities.

### Amount and type of practice
It has been a long-held maxim that practice is a major variable in the acquisition of a motor skill, both the amount of practice and the structure of the practice. However it is probably the amount of *appropriate* practice that is of most importance. There is evidence to show that performance can be characterized by jumps, plateaus and even decrements in performance.

Schmidt and Lee (2011, p. 286) state, 'Clearly more learning will occur if there are more practice trials, all other things being equal.'

It is debatable whether it is deliberate practice or exposure and experience with a known aim and a number of variables that contribute to this process. There are various learning curves (see Chapter 2) but the one that is most common is the negatively accelerated curve, with more gains in performance at the beginning of the learning period and the gains gradually becoming less as practice continues. Thus, the amount and type of practice is what the teacher and therapist will need to consider carefully.

The amount of practice required is linked to how the child is participating, and so the variables that contribute to participation need to be considered. Very often the level participation is in the hands of the professional, not the child. At the macro level within society, to the micro level in the classroom or clinical setting, the context can be modified to suit the resources of the child, thereby facilitating participation and the practice that follows.

*Distribution of practice*
It is often said that little and often describes how much each practice session should contain and how often it ought to take place. Throughout the book we have emphasized the idea of making many small modifications to the child's life. The accumulation of marginal gains in many areas generates bigger improvement overall. Some modifications take place all the time so that the child is constantly changing their activities of daily living. However, sometimes formal practice needs to be provided. This is a continuum of experience and practice. Continued improvement has face validity in other arenas, such as the sport and music. This informal practice can be built into everyday life.

In a formal practice situation, for a child with handwriting difficulties for example, a face valid assumption would be that it is better to have 15 to 20 minutes practice every day as than 40 to 50 minutes once or twice a week. From a motivational point of view it is much easier to keep children, especially young ones, motivated for a short rather than a long period of time. In addition, with short sessions, the work becomes more easily part of the child's daily routine; it blends into all activities of daily living and is not seen as a one-off session to be endured. This is particularly true if the child is working in collaboration with a professional.

While this makes intuitive sense, the question is, does one practice protocol show any advantage over the other? Again, much will depend on the task, whether it is discrete, serial or continuous and also the environmental context in which the skill is to be learned and executed. When applying the principles of motor learning to populations of children with a range of motor and behavioural challenges, it is important to proceed with caution with regard to the strict, application of the motor learning principles discussed here. This is because specific clinical populations may not respond in the same way, as suggested by extant research, which has been conducted mainly on typical young adults.

*Blocked, serial and random practice*
When organizing practice, intuitively an instructor might reason that focused practice is required to achieve a necessary skill level. Thus, practice variability (see Chapter 2)

and the introduction of 'contextual interference' into the practice schedule become important variables. In Chapter 2, we described three separate learning to walk scenarios: a *blocked* schedule in which the individual practices one scenario before going to the next; a *serial* schedule where the learner practices a combination of the three scenarios in order; and a *random* schedule, a scenario whereby each of the three versions of walking are presented in a random order, so that each scenario could not be anticipated by the learner.

The random presentation challenges the learner and would seem to slow the rate of learning at the beginning , which could lead to frustration in a child with movement difficulties. However, it does have the advantage of being flexible in dealing with unexpected events. Clinical and professional experience leans towards a modified practice protocol that requires first blocked practice to learn the skill and provide motivation, followed by serial practice, using random practice as a long-term objective.

### Variability of practice
Ever since Schmidt published his famous article on schema learning in 1975, there has been considerable debate about the **variability of practice.** We have noted that a child in a learning situation requires a variability of response to meet changing environmental circumstances. The variability of practice, or schema learning, has face validity to achieve this end and produce a schema that can generate functional movements for a particular class of events. According to this theory, there exist generalized motor programmes for each task that can be applied to a wide range of tasks, rather than having separate motor programmes for each task.

The empirical literature supporting schema theory is equivocal. Most of the studies examining this working use experimental tasks in narrow laboratory-based settings. Davids et al. (2008) notes that a number of factors mediate the potential benefits of variable practice, such as the age of the participants, with younger children seeming to benefit more than adults. The available literature suggests that both ballistic and complex skills are helped by variable practice.

Schmidt (1975) advanced the thinking in this field in a considerably. Many studies have tested the theory of variability of practice and related issues, and it has been taken up globally by practitioners. Despite some misgivings, it is an important and influential theory and there is some evidence of its effectiveness in children (Kerr and Booth 1978; Shapiro and Schmidt 1982; Green et al. 1995). It also works together with the concept of variability we discuss later in this chapter.

The general rule is that the conditions and tasks in training should match those that are going to be required in everyday life. They should provide flexibility to approach and perform a range of tasks. This is why we favour task-oriented approaches, which are directly concerned with activities of daily living as opposed to underlying processes that often seem divorced from objective. Learning becomes more complicated when tasks are broken down in to their component parts, which is an often-used strategy in task-based approaches. Again, the relationship between the individual parts and the finished and desired task should be as close as possible.

It is not only the evidence from a specific task, but the context in which each task is performed. Thus, the wider context such as school or home will all have an effect on the learning process. In the first instance, these should be as constant and similar as possible and then as the individual becomes more proficient, they can be extended and varied so that when a child approaches a novel situation, he or she has a repertoire of skills to approach and solve the problem.

In handwriting, for example, the child could be to asked to write as fast as they can, present their neatest writing, copy from a whiteboard, trace, or listen to instructions and write them down. Other manual tasks would include in-hand manipulation, using fingers to manipulate such items as coins; reaching and grasping for objects using the hand and arm or gripping tightly to generate force, such as in using a hammer.

*Mental practice*
Much of the evidence for the efficacy mental practice comes from either group laboratory experiments or from individual accounts of mental practice in a game situation, particularly in sport. The experimental work in this area involves quite complex conditions comprising no practice, practice on an unrelated task, practice on the actual task, mental practice and variations on all of these. Often in controlled experiments on mental practice there are up to 12 groups working under a variety of conditions trying to tease out its effects.

Overall, the evidence shows that, under comparable conditions, physical practice is preferable and more advantageous than mental practice. (Schmidt and Lee 2011). However, where physical practice is not available or possible, mental practice can be effective in providing a learning experience to the individual such as the mental processes required to execute complex tasks that require a sequence of activities. Schmidt and Lee (2011) note that other possibilities include implicit speech, which involves individuals imagining the movement that may trigger internal mechanisms such as the Golgi tendon organs; spindle mechanisms, or feed-forward movements that are generated when motor programmes are in operation. They conclude that planning, itself a mental process, is beneficial to learning but that little evidence is available to distinguish between the various types of mental processes.

*Meaningful and enjoyable*
When a child is practicing a particular skill, there is more likelihood of success if the task is meaningful and enjoyable to the child; hopefully this is what the child

encounters in everyday life. The child can engage in both informal and formal practices: on their own children can practice skills informally during the course of daily living such as keeping a diary or texting. More formal practices would include making games out of practice sessions and setting targets for friendly non-threatening competition. Letting the child choose many of the activities, and charting the results are all ways in which tasks can be made more enjoyable. For example, if throwing is involved, the child should throw at targets; if it is a writing exercise, the child could develop his own story or make his or her own stencils. The teachers should encourage practice in a way that leads eventually to good performance in daily life situations and provide a clear structure, which provides the child with the stability he or she needs to take command of the learning situation.

When the task is complete, plenty of praise should be given and it should be clear what the praise is for. For example, 'Well done Amy, your writing is much better now that you are sitting correctly and you worked hard'. This is more appropriate than just 'Good girl, Amy'. In the former Amy knows what she has done and why, whereas in the latter she simply knows she is a good girl, which could apply to anything. Activities that are meaningful and intrinsically enjoyable for the child are much more likely to enable the child to be fully engaged.

When a child fails on a regular basis the solution might to change the attributions the child uses as to why they fail. In attribution theory, a child who fails regularly usually ascribes the failure to ability, and if successful, attributes the cause to luck or the task being easy. A successful child ascribes success to ability and hard work and failure to not trying hard enough. The lesson from this is that we should encourage children by teaching them that hard work will produce success, even if it is slow in coming, and not ascribe success or failure to luck, task difficulty or ability.

*Goal setting*

Studies on adults show that specific set goals of moderate difficulty are better than those that are vague or too ambitious. It is also useful to differentiate between short and long-term goals, particularly when asking children what they would like to achieve. Short-term goals may include the next practice session or two, such as learning to catch a small ball while running, with a longer-term goal would be being an active participant in peer-related ball games. Research has also shown us that, at different stages of the learning process, the importance of particular goals may change. The CanChild team have developed a system involving goal setting called the Perceived Efficacy and Goal Setting (PEGS) (Missiuna et al. 2004) that enables young children (ages 5–9y) to self-report their perceived competence in everyday activities and to set goals for intervention. The children use a set of cards showing self-care, school and leisure activities, and choose which are challenging for them and which ones they would like to work on.

*Expert scaffolding*

We use the term expert scaffolding (from Vygotsky's Zone of Proximal Development [ZOPD] 1978), to describe the process by which a more accomplished person such as a parent supports to the child to ensure initial success and gradually withdraws it so the child can manage their own learning. This support or 'scaffolding' can take many forms: support whereby the parent (sometimes passively such as using an arm) guides the child; support by breaking the task into smaller parts, as in task analysis and then building it back up; support by simplifying the whole task and then making it more complex; or support by changing the environmental demands by making it easier and more motivating. Thus, support can be the adding of something more detailed or complex or the withdrawing of support, such that the child is taking more control and responsibility for their own learning.

*Problem-solving strategies*

With many motor challenges, there is no set way to accomplish the task. Someone can pick up a paper in many different ways, or catch a ball with one hand or two hands. A ball can be thrown overhand or underhand, with one or two hands, or with a bounce. An individual can climb stairs taking them one at a time or bound up them two or three at time.

The way we solve these challenges again depends on the context, something we have stressed throughout this book. The interaction between the resources of the individual and the environmental demands will guide how the task is dealt with. For example, when hitting a golf ball into the wind, or kicking a soccer ball on a wet muddy surface, the environmental conditions will be an important consideration to ensure a successful outcome. Using problem-solving strategies is at the heart of some programmes (Henderson and Sugden 1992), including the very popular CO-OP programme (Polatajko et al. 2001). In addition, the individual seeking solutions to the contextual situation is what is called non-linear pedagogies, which advocate discovery learning, where the individual is actively engaged in seeking functional answers to a particular movement situation (Davids et al. 2008). In the first instance, this exploratory behaviour helps the individual create the coordination patterns to achieve a particular task and with progression, facilitates refining and adapting to achieve flexibility of response to meet changing contextual circumstances (Davids et al. 2003).

*Knowing and doing – planning and execution*

When a child has a movement difficulty it can be for a variety of reasons. If we broadly split task performance into 'knowing' and 'doing' or 'planning' and 'executing', some children have difficulty with one or both parts.

A coordination difficulty is a doing activity (knowing how), whereas just knowing is really only setting the scene. It is our opinion that for too long we have concentrated on the 'knowing' part of a skill, such as executive function, and not enough on the coordination or the 'doing' part. We recognize that a child with known planning difficulties will need activities that increase the level of difficulty both for decision-making and the sequencing of activities. Use of visual and other cues can help here, such as footprints to step into for the child planning where he or she ought to go in navigating a course. However, the doing part or coordination needs substantial support for the child to acquire a range of skills that can adapt to changing environmental demands.

*Changing associated behaviours*
We have noted that children with movement problems often have associated difficulties. These can be with attention, anti-social behaviours or simply that they move too fast, too often and at the wrong time. Attention may be difficult for them; picking out the relevant features of a task tests them and staying on task is often nearly impossible. For example, a child may be impulsive, disruptive, overestimate their own ability, or simply be overactive. Their movement skills may not be poor but their behaviour is sometimes overwhelming. It is important to go to the core of the problem (attentional difficulties), and then consider the multidimensionality of this important variable. For example, attention issues can involve coming to attention, selective attention, impulsivity, persistence and freedom from distractibility, all requiring different strategies. If the child is impulsive or overactive it is important to present activities that require planning for their success; activities that need to be performed in a controlled manner and activities that are performed slowly. Tracing a line slowly, balancing a bean-bag on the head while walking on a line, balancing a ball on a book while zig-zag walking in and out of cones, are activities that can be employed.

*Instructions, demonstrations and feedback*
A major point in motor learning and practice is the influence of instructions, demonstrations and feedback. We have noted that at various stages of the learning process these will differ, ranging from simple instructions to enable the individual to practice the task to more complex ones as they become more proficient.

From a dynamic constraints viewpoint, the aim of these variables is to aid the individual's search for optimum solutions to the task at hand. Proponents of this approach emphasize the effect of the movement on the external environment rather than on the internal movement dynamics. Focusing on the movement effects provides better opportunities for individuals to learn the range of opportunities that are present in a task-context situation. Davids et al. (2003) provides examples in volley-ball and tennis of how concentrating on the movement effects on the environment, promotes more effective learning. When providing feedback, concentrating too much on the movement dynamics, that is form and technique, can hinder the acquisition of flexible and adaptive learning. Box 6.5 shows the variables that could be considered when organizing practice for learning motor skills.

**Box 6.5** Variables that affect motor learning and practice

- ✓ Amount and type of practice
- ✓ Distribution of practice
- ✓ Variability of practice-structure
- ✓ Practice and specificity
- ✓ Mental practice
- ✓ Meaningful and enjoyable activities
- ✓ Goal setting
- ✓ Expert scaffolding
- ✓ Problem solving strategies
- ✓ Knowing and doing
- ✓ Changing associated behaviours
- ✓ Instructions, demonstrations and feedback

## From specific skills to generalization

*Learning specific skills*

Very often we find that an individual has to learn a specific skill by being taught directly. This could be, for example, tying shoelaces, riding a bicycle or making handwriting more legible. To do this, therapists, teachers and parents engage in the practice of task analysis and task adaptation. Both of these activities combine and interact in a dynamic manner to help the child both participate and learn the new skill.

*Task adaptation*

The adaptation of a task involves changing the presentation of the task to make it easier for the child to participate. By participating more, the child will have more time on task, which is an important variable for learning and performance. Two examples of task adaptation are shown in Figure 6.2.

In physical education lessons can require movement from one place to another, by running, jumping, hopping skipping. The choice of these activities can be left to the individual child. The child could be asked, 'See how many different ways you can move from a to using your legs and arms'. The child can then choose the level of difficulty that is commensurate with their ability and the teacher can suggest more complex ways when the child has mastered their initial choice.

*Task analysis*

Here the task is broken down into its component parts such that the child can achieve each part. The parts are sequenced in such a way that he or she can place them together

### 1. Rules of a game change

If a child has difficulty striking a ball thrown, in a game such as softball, the ball can be placed on top of a cone and struck while it is stationary. If the fielding side has difficulty in throwing and catching the ball, the game can be modified such that they have to run to the cone and place the ball back on it before the batter gets back. Different rules can be inserted such as the ball must pass through more than one person before being placed on the cone, according to the ability of the children. Ball games such as this can be modified in many different ways.

### 2. Writing and drawing implements (pens and pencils change)

There are now many different pens, pencils, felt-tips etc. that present a variety of grips and tips that can accommodate most hands and grip styles. These include writing implements with different shapes and weights, with soft grips in various materials. Examples can be found at https://www.thedyslexiashop.co.uk/stationery-for-dyslexics/pens-pencils-and-writing-aids.html.

### 3. Different types of keyboards

Larger keyboards –up to 4x size. Ranges of mice that are easier to grip and control.

### 4. Modification of equipment for more gross motor skills

- For ball games:
  Balls of different shapes and sizes (see a); bean-bags; velcro balls and mitts for catching; bigger and lighter rackets and sticks for tennis and hockey; scoops for catching in general, batting tees (see b).

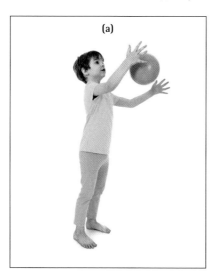 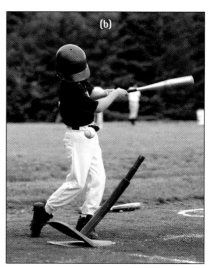

(a) Catching a large ball; (b) striking off a tee – this could also be a cone if a tee is not available.

- For balance and agility:
  Different shapes and lengths and widths of balance beams; climbing apparatus that can be adjusted to the ability of the children; boards and disks for balance and adjustable.

Much equipment that is found in regular schools can be adapted to the needs of the children. It is also recommended that readers consult the commercial sites that produce these products.

**Figure 6.2** Task adaptation.

> **Box 6.6** Task analysis of bicycle riding (Dunford et al. 2016)
>
> 1. Child puts on helmet
> 2. Child mounts and dismounts the stationary cycle
> 3. Pedals taken off the cycle and child scoots the cycle with feet
> 4. Pedals off the bike and child brakes to command
> 5. Pedals off the bike and child scoots and steers in and out of cones
> 6. Pedals on the bike and child pedals with safety belt short distance
> 7. Pedals on the bike and child with safety harness and brakes to command
> 8. Pedals on the bike and child with safety harness steers in an out of cones
> 9. No safety harness and child repeats 5, 6 and 7

with ease into the required whole. The challenge for the teacher, therapist or parent is to ensure that the sequence of events is correct in terms of the breakdown, the number of steps and how they come back into a whole. If there are too many parts to the analysis, then the whole may be a distant vision. If the steps are too large, then the child may have difficulty in moving from one to another. A basic example of task analysis of cycle riding is shown in Box 6.6.

This can all be broken down in much more detail and modified with more advanced practices, according to context and child's rate of learning and ability. The task is being simplified with 'riding' still predominating.

In other tasks ,such as volley-ball or serving in tennis, Davids et al. (2003) recommend **task simplification** rather than **task decomposition.** Thus, in tennis the toss of the ball to serve should not be decoupled from the strike with the racket but instead simplified. This is an important point as it keeps the practice functional and recognized by the learner. The starting point could be with the racket already placed in the ready position 'scratching the back' and the serve takes place accordingly and is not simply practicing tossing the ball then swiping at an imaginary ball as independent actions. Our view is that simplification or decoupling depends on the nature of the task and, as far as possible, the conditions of practice reflecting what will be required in the actual game situation.

Many of these are described and elaborated later in this chapter and in more detail in the Case Studies in Chapter 7.

### Teaching for generalization
The transfer and generalization of skills to different situations is a concept that has attracted substantial research in the motor learning literature, mainly in adults. Schmidt and Lee (2011) outline a number of principles germane to the concept. Two principles stand out: (1) the amount of transfer is positive but small unless tasks are very similar and (2) the amount of

transfer depends upon the similarity of the tasks. Transfer from one task to a totally different activity, what Schmidt and Lee (2011) call inter-task transfer is small or negligible.

One could view **task analysis** as **involving transfer,** with the task broken down into its components parts for practice, anticipating transfer to the whole. The evidence appears to be good for this when the task is complex, but sometimes it is difficult to reassemble the parts because of the temporal organization (sequencing and timing) of the task. Simulation has been used for transfer in the form of virtual reality, and although it is at the early stages of capturing evidence for this group of approaches, it appears to be a promising avenue.

Despite reservations about the total effectiveness of these approaches to teaching for transfer, it is something we must engage in because there is insufficient time to teach directly all the skills that are required by children with movement difficulties. Later in this chapter we outline the ways in which the optimal levels of transfer can be achieved.

### Variations of tasks

More often than not we are required to use skills in novel and different situations and contexts. If we have only been taught to be consistent with our response then there is the danger that when adaptability and flexibility is required we are not equipped to meet this demand. Consistency may be desirable in simple, closed tasks but if the context is changing or different demands are made then flexibility of response is required. Modifications to accommodate variability and facilitate flexibility are shown in Box 6.7.

Tasks can be grouped according to the part of the body used, outcome, environmental condition or a combination of all three. The term **manual control** is a general movement classification for arm and hand movements used to control objects. One can consider the **hand as a unit** focusing on the movements of the five digits for **grasp and manipulation**. This can involve such activities such as turning a coin in the hand, or simply holding a pencil. Figure 6.3 illustrates the various grips young children use when painting.

---

**Box 6.7** Variability of tasks

✓ Slightly modifying the task to a changing/moving context rather than a static one, different speed and force requirements.

✓ Performing the task with someone other than the usual instructor/parent, etc.

✓ Performing the task in a totally different place – school, home, workplace.

✓ Performing the task with different equipment (ball catching, bean bag, small ball, large playground ball; different sizes of buttons to fasten, etc.).

---

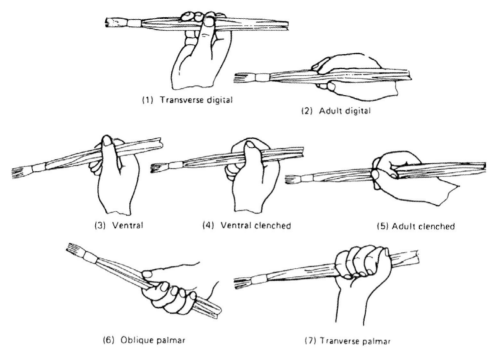

(1) Transverse digital

(2) Adult digital

(3) Ventral          (4) Ventral clenched          (5) Adult clenched

(6) Oblique palmar          (7) Transverse palmar

**Figure 6.3** Grip variations of 3- and 4-year-old children when painting on an upright easel.

Source: Connolly and Elliott (1972). Reproduced with permission.

As can be seen in Box 6.8, moving the hand, however, is a **function for the arm** that also provides **support and transport** and indeed a **modulation of force,** such as when using a hammer. Other simple activities involve reaching for an object and picking it up. The arm is transporting the hand to the correct position and the fingers then close

---

**Box 6.8** Generic manual functions

*The hand can*
✓ Grasp and manipulate
✓ Be used uni- or bimanually

*The arm can*
✓ Support and transport
✓ Modulate force

*The arm and hand together can*
✓ Produce continuous and serial movements
✓ Receive and intercept moving objects
✓ Produce gestures, e.g. thumbs up

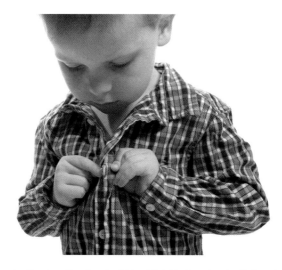

**Figure 6.4** A young boy buttoning the front of his shirt. He is using both hands and the buttons are visible.

in with appropriate spacing and timing on the object. A third group involves **serial or continuous movements,** such as writing and drawing. A final group is based on **receiving and intercepting moving objects,** such as catching, meeting or avoiding other moving objects with the hand and arm.

The first of our functions involves a group based upon actions such as turning a coin in the hand or opening a wallet or buttoning a shirt. Some of these are unimanual, such as the coin turning, others are bimanual such as buttoning a shirt (see Fig. 6.4). These can be labelled as **manipulation.** These activities have common features such as the movements being typically intrinsic, within the hand and using much kinaesthetic information (Elliott and Connolly 1972; Connolly and Elliott 1974). These movements can be regarded as part of the same **class of events.** Thus, in order to cater for the range in this class of events, variable practice is given to include as many available movements as possible. In addition, variable practice would enable the individual to approach a novel movement with confidence. Tasks that involved, press-studs, laces, or zippers, could be included in this form of variable practice. Where progression is involved, there may be movement from unimanual to bimanual manipulation, depending on the task. Although there will be some visual guidance occurring, much of it is kinaesthetically driven.

A second part of manual skills involves **reaching and grasping** and this group provides another class of events. Here the child is often reaching to pick up an object, either with one hand or two. Research has shown that there are two basic components in this task:

the first is the transport of the hand and arm to the appropriate position and the second is the progressive closing of the hand and fingers with the grip appropriate to the size of the object. This is a different class of events from manipulation as the action is very much visually guided. Different sized and shaped objects are used at different distances to help the child develop a series of reaching and grasping responses, and known and new objects can be engaged. The child is to be encouraged to discover the various ways in which the task can be accomplished with an emphasis on the environmental effect rather than on a strict technique.

A third group of manual skills would involve **serial and continuous movements** such as drawing, writing and copying. The child is constantly uses on-going feedback to alter and modify the action so that the writing is legible, and so on. These are not in the same grouping/class of activities as the first two groups of manual skills (see Box 6.9), yet many of the same principles may apply. Such things as letter and word formation are constant but the child could be asked to copy, or freely write or write slowly or quickly. This variation in output can provide a class of events that the child can use in different and novel situations. The above three types of movements are examples of how varying the practice sessions can help. Some tasks lend themselves to 'wider' or 'narrower' classes of events and the child is encouraged to find their own solutions to these.

A final group involves **intercepting moving objects** with the hand and arm. This can involve catching objects or striking moving objects such as in games like softball. Initially for catching a ball, the hand has to be placed in the correct position using the arm to intercept the ball and then the hand has to close around the ball with precise timing. Striking an object is different in that the hand remains stable around an implement such as a bat, and it is the arm that is producing the exact movement, although the hand does 'tweak' the bat or racket in some instances, such as tennis.

---

**Box 6.9** Task variations of manual skills

*Manipulation: Intrinsic movements with one hand*

*Intrinsic movements two hands*
- ✓ Coin turning, button fastening, threading laces and beads, zippers, velcro, snaps

*Reaching and grasping and letting go*
- ✓ Reaching to pick up a pencil

*Serial and continuous movements*
- ✓ Writing, drawing, tracing and copying

*Receiving objects to intercept and catch, strike or avoid*
- ✓ Different balls, distances, trajectory, force

---

> **Box 6.10** Guidelines for generalization
>
> ✓ It is helpful if the child is able to accomplish all of the component parts that the therapist/teacher has presented.
> ✓ The gaps between the component parts should not be so broad that the child cannot discover and easily recognize the seamless sequence between them.
> ✓ The task should not be broken down into so many small parts that the overall task is lost. The task should remain meaningful.

### *Learner action*

Another way in which a child can be helped to achieve transfer to a wider variety of skills is via their own actions and problem solving. Here we are looking at some of the cognitive aspects of a task and what they involve, which may help the production of movement flexibility.

There have been a number of approaches based on this maxim, such as the cognitive motor approach by Henderson and Sugden (1992), ecological intervention (Sugden and Henderson 2007) and the now widely used CO-OP approach (Polatajko and Mandich 2004).

*Child Task Analysis.* One of the activities that all good clinicians and teachers engage in is to analyse the task to determine first, what it involves for the child and second, to break it down into smaller components that can eventually be combined into the whole task. There are a number of guidelines for doing this. Box 6.10 provides guidelines to aid **generalization**.

One of the assets that skilled learners have is to be able to break down tasks themselves. We are not suggesting that the child does all of this but as it is the aim of the therapist to withdraw from the learning process part of this involves transferring part of the onus of learning the task onto the child. The aim is to enable the child to become an independent learner such that he or she can operate without instruction in everyday life. Thus, the first part of this sequence is all important: 'What does the task require of me? What is it asking me to do? Are there any things in my skill repertoire that can help me with this task?' These questions are part of the transfer process it. This will help in the transfer and generalization of any skill. To aid in this process the teacher/therapist may use these assisted questions, following the Vygotsky line of Zone of Proximal Development, where the potential of the child is the difference between what they can achieve on their own and what they can accomplish with the help of a more capable other. Thus, the assisted questions can help the child learn to problem solve. This is where process and task approaches overlap. We are teaching a child to be competent in a number of tasks and are teaching the task directly, but we are assisting this direct teaching by asking the

> **Box 6.11** The essence of our approach to intervention in a child with movement difficulties
>
> *Evidence from theory, empiricism and professional practice*
>
> *Individual profile with objectives*
>
> *Multiple inputs to programme priorities*
> ✓ Child, parents, teachers, health, others
>
> *Graded approach*
> ✓ In class to all children; small group teaching; individual tuition
>
> *Group teaching*
> ✓ All children on similar programme to ensure participation
>
> *Individual tuition*
> ✓ To direct to specific individual needs of child
>
> *Different partners contributing to programme enactment*
> ✓ School, home, health, community

child to use cognitive processes to tackle the task. Box 6.11 summarizes our approach to intervention principles.

A key feature of our approach is that every child is a unique individual and although there are general principles that will apply to all children, the specific needs, strengths and weaknesses of each child should be directly addressed.

The approach is a graded one that moves from generic teaching for all children through to specific and detailed support and intervention for those who require it. Thus, we would always start with all children being given the opportunity to participate and learn a whole variety of movement skills. This can be done in the classroom at home and in the community.

All children are presented with movement challenges to solve. Those that show difficulties are moved through a series of options involving changing the task, or the context to make them more accessible with varying degrees of increased support that gradually become more detailed. A variety of approaches are used, utilizing group teaching and individual tuition and therapy.

We believe that the evidence for **teaching of functional skills** is valid, reliable and secure and we will present various methods to do this. One could argue that when teaching functional skills and using cognitive problem solving strategies we are also invoking underlying processes and most importantly engineering the environment so that the environmental context affords an appropriate response. In this way the child is never the unit of an analysis – it is always the child in context.

This approach is set in a much wider approach about movements being taught in context. The process involves both **participation and learning (**see Chapter 5**)**. We noted in earlier chapters that learning rarely occurs without participation and in order to bring about increased participation, we have to make adjustments to the context and the wider environment. By making the environment more inviting (and affording participation), we are providing the foundations for improved learning. This in turn allows the child to exploit their own resources and increases the types of environments in which the child can participate. he result is an upward moving cycle of improvement. We should not over emphasize the time spent on any task, for although it is important, it is just one variable that moves the skill level upwards. What children do during practice is crucial, and we have always maintained that it is the amount and the appropriateness of the practice that are the important variables.

An often quoted example is of the person with apraxia who has difficulty in translating a verbal command into a required action: the therapist asks the person to wave; the young man with apraxia cannot do this. The therapist then asks him to imitate her waving, again he cannot do this. She then says that she will see him in a week's time and as he leaves the room he waves goodbye. The movement is now in context; leaving the room sets up an environmental affordance that invites waving. The young man had no need to abstract a context, which could not do with the first two requests. The power of context can often moderate a supposed neurological deficit.

## How should we teach?

Much of what we have covered so far has been derived from well-honed and researched studies in the area of motor learning. While much of it is traditional literature, more recently, many researchers and practitioners have added to this work by invoking the dynamic systems approach to learning and performance. Much of this we covered in Chapters 2 and 5 and we believe that a combination of these two approaches can be best utilized for an optimum effect on children's motor learning. **A combination of traditional motor learning practices together with dynamic systems approaches appears to be the most favourable approach.**

A traditional approach has involved the teacher/therapist giving practice sessions to try to perfect a performance and carefully manage the learning situation, such as in physical education or a clinical session.

Teaching Games for Understanding (Bunker and Thorpe 1982; Thorpe 1990; Gallwey 2015); the Inner Game series (Chow et al. 2006); constraints led skill acquisition (Davids et al. 2003), non-linear pedagogies (Davids et al. 2008) and ecological intervention (Sugden and Henderson 2007).

Our teaching and therapy, therefore, is based upon the following guidelines.

First, we work with the **child in context** with this dynamic being the unit of analysis. It is constraints led with the constraints of **task, environment and the child resources** all playing an interacting dynamical role. This is the basis of our work, with modifications to the context and the environment, all feeding back and forth into a changing child resources scenario.

**Different individuals will provide different levels of support** at various times and locations. This specialist support from therapists and others is cascaded to parents, teachers, and the child such that small gains are made with only slight modifications to the child's daily routine.

Skills are built into the fabric of daily life through specialist advice to those who see the child on a regular basis.

**Individual goal setting is recommended.** This does not mean that the child is taught individually, as we believe group teaching fosters other qualities besides improvement in motor skills. However, goal setting is tailored to the needs and wishes of the child. Individual goal setting is recommended but taught in small group situations.

Therapy/teaching should be based on **real life situations** not laboratory based or involving merely the repetition of movements. These real life situations can be varied to encourage flexible responses to a movement problem. We know from various sources that practice involves 'variety-practice', which is defined as repetition without repetition (Bernstein 1967). A similar paraphrase comes from Bartlett (1932): when we practice a task we never do something completely different nor do we simply repeat our movements. We are looking for functional variability where we can perform different actions to achieve the same functional end result.

We utilize the time honoured **principles of motor learning** described earlier in the chapter on distribution of practice, time on task, specificity of practice, mental practice, contextual interference, feedback schedules, and associated behaviours, and so on. The recommendations from studies on these variables have been quite robust over a number of years. But what we are less sure of is how they apply to children and young adults with movement difficulties. How we present the learning situations, structure practice, provide instructions, demonstrations and feedback is crucial aspects of the learning process and have well-established evidence.

**Solving a movement problem is the outcome,** not one that is predetermined. In this way, the individual is better equipped to deal with the novel movement challenges that are present in everyday life. Thus, dynamic answers to a movement problem are temporally assembled according to contextual demand and child resources. Teaching games for understanding, constraint-led skill acquisition and non-linear pedagogies are examples of this type of approach.

Movement solutions are often temporary and transient, but will be recruited specifically for solving a current movement problem. As solutions are often temporary it follows that therapeutic practices should not aim for a predetermined action; flexible functional solutions are required.

**Associated personal characteristics** such as psycho-social aspects, self-concept and self-esteem should always be considered. These are variables that will affect the type of support and intervention that is provided.

A child with a low self-concept will require a modification of support, compared with one who has a good level of resilience.

If a child has a **low standard of fitness in strength, endurance or flexibility**, remedying this should be built into the support programme. It may be done in a skilled manner at the same time as the coordination issues are being addressed.

We recognize that both **development and learning are non-linear**. Learning, we recognize, does not progress in a smooth regular fashion. It often moves in steps, like jumps, then often plateaus and occasionally has decrements. Thus, if a skill is being learned there may be rapid learning in the first instance, then a slowing down in what we know as a negatively accelerated learning curve. Big gains are present early on with smaller gains later. Similarly, if we examine development we see parallel trends (see Fig. 3.5).

From this we look to the different stages of learning and/or development to modify our instructions, demonstrations and feedback.

**Variability can be reduced or increased to environmental task demand**. If the task requires consistency as in a 'closed' task such as the formation of letters, we look to reduce variability. However, in an open task, such as ball catching, we may need to increase variability or flexibility so that the individual has the resources to adapt to the changing contextual circumstances. More often than not, variability of response is to be celebrated rather than looked on as something that ought to be reduced. If one takes a crude approach to variability one can say that in any atypical population, the variability between and within individuals is invariably higher than that in a typically developed, matched population. However, this view of variability assumes that it is bad to have high variability. This is not always, or even often, the case, as we are looking for adaptability and flexibility much of the time, so that the learner is able to respond to an increasingly complex and changing dynamic situation. Reducing variability of response is not always the answer and what is required will be a function of contextual demand. Increasing flexibility of response is often necessary to answer a changing context and practice should reflect this. A crucial point is that variability in any task should be recognized by the learner as useful and not as something that is error laden. Variability in movement (enhanced flexibility) can be seen as of great value in the learning process (Smith et al. 2015). Sport has numerous examples of individuals who perform with unique and unusual methods. Davids et al. (2008, p. 52) make a good point when they say: 'Variation permits a flexible adaptation, the constraints of a dynamic environment, a useful characteristic in rich and diverse performance contexts.'

There may be **specific skills that are deficient,** such as handwriting, and if so, a programme directly aimed at this is required. It may be that, at the same time, keyboard skills are addressed, if it is felt necessary.

Both learning and development are the outcomes from a **self-organizing system** that has constraints that act to create a dynamic system. Thelen (1995) notes that when systems self-organize they create states that are 'comfortable', this mode being called an attractor state. When the system is just slightly perturbed, it can maintain its preferred state. Bigger fluctuations around stable states are the sources of new behaviours and development. To some extent this is an unpredictable situation.

We often say that appropriate action involves both **knowing and doing.** However, in most situations that children with movement difficulties face it is the 'doing' that is important for the smooth coordination of the output. The 'knowing' does not come from within in a cognitive manner but is embedded in the environmental context, with the affordances present inviting the appropriate action. For example, Newell has shown that simply by altering the size of cubes, infants will automatically switch from one handed to two handed grasping. Similarly, I noticed that my granddaughter at 10 months used a crude palmar grasp to pick up peas that are in a bunch, but switches to a pincer grip when they are placed one by one in a line. Box 6.12 summarizes the approach we take to teaching motor skills.

Many times we have presented our model of the process that involves the task the environment and the learner resources. The transactions between these three components change throughout the learning process in a non-linear dynamic fashion. There are 'jumps' to more mature patterns of motor behaviour with periods of stability, which may then be upset by instability requiring a 'jump' to another state.

> **Box 6.12** How should we teach motor skills?
>
> ✓ Child in context – ecological Intervention
> ✓ Different individuals providing different levels of support
> ✓ Individual goal setting
> ✓ Real life situations
> ✓ Solving a movement problem
> ✓ Principles of motor learning
> ✓ Associated personal characteristics
> ✓ Fitness, if necessary
> ✓ Non-linear development and learning
> ✓ Increase or reduce variability, according to task demands
> ✓ Self-organizing system
> ✓ Knowing and doing

Davids et al. (2008) include many of these guidelines in their work on non-linear pedagogies and how they are enacted in practice. Below we present summaries of two of their case study examples, followed by how this approach is implemented in our case studies. We would supplement these by utilizing the guidelines on practice schedules and presentation from the traditional motor learning literature (Davids et al. 2008).

*Case study example 1: Soccer chip*
Keith Davids has been a good soccer player and it is not surprising to find the skill of chipping a ball in his book. The book describes an example of a woman soccer player whose coordination patterns are not good. Her non-kicking foot being too far away from the ball together with too much leaning back of upper body. In a typical coaching situation, the coach would probably address the player directly, asking her to place her foot nearer the ball and not lean back too much. Here the decision was taken to manipulate the task constraints, not the player, and directly address the task. A 1-metre high barrier was placed 2 metres away from the player and the player was asked to alternatively pass the ball under and over the barrier. The coach here is manipulating the task constraints so that the player will search from the available environmental information (affordance) for the appropriate body position and foot placements for successful task completion. After a few attempts, a team-mate was placed behind the barrier and the player was asked to pass the ball to him acting as a receiver. Again, with little instruction the player is searching for the appropriate solution to the task. This continued with more advanced challenges, such as kicking the ball to the receiver and then moving to receive, as well as changing the barrier heights. The player is invited

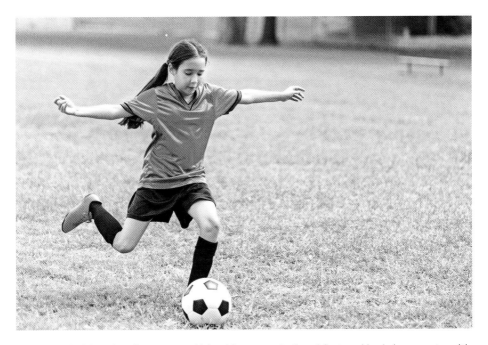

**Figure 6.5** A girl performing a soccer kick with eyes on ball and foot and body in correct position.

to respond to the affordances in the environment in order to find the appropriate solution. Little instruction, if any, is given about how to do this with the player being encouraged to search for the solution within the task constraints that are provided. Figure 6.5 shows a girl performing a soccer kick with eyes on ball and foot and body in the correct position.

*Case study example 2: Disability*
Two patients with transtibial amputations had the aim of walking as soon as possible. Both had prosthetics and attempted to walk measured on a treadmill (see Fig. 6.6). One adapted to the prosthesis better than the other, probably due to being fitter as he had worked as a mail delivery person for 8 years. The other had a more sedentary office job. Obstacles were placed on the floor for them to walk over and the fitter patient completed the route quicker than the other patient, but made more mistakes. The other patient took longer but took bigger strides. For the patient who made more mistakes, the task was modified with a rope ladder placed on the floor asking him to walk accurately in the gaps. This task constraint facilitated more accurate walking while keeping the speed at a good pace. For the other patient, conditioning exercises were recommended so that he could make the strides more quickly. This example shows, again, that modifying the task constraints affords different solutions and that these solutions will differ according to the constraint of the person resources.

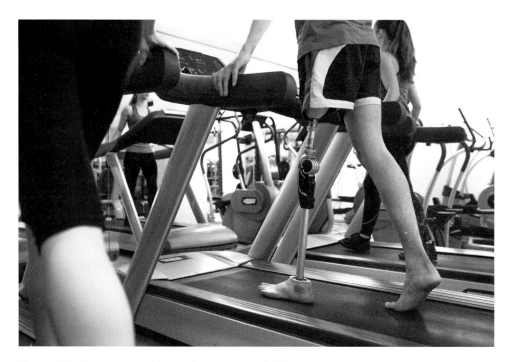

**Figure 6.6** Amputee practicing walking on a treadmill.

In both of these examples Davids et al. (2008) are stressing that the doing of an action is the important part. Any knowing part is done with respect to the outcome of the task by a problem-solving route that will be unique to the individual mover and does not need to be verbalized or even be made aware of. It is a match between the environmental demand and the resources of the individual, where the coordination for that particular act is temporarily ('softly') assembled according to the affordances the environment.

*Case study example 3: Tennis serve*

This example of Davids et al. (2008) is one that one of the authors (Sugden) is familiar with having been a tennis coach. The usual method of teaching a tennis serve is to note that it has two parts – accurate tossing of the ball and then instructions like 'Throw the racket head at the ball' or other phrases that try to encapsulate the serving action often, with a correct technique being the goal (see Fig. 6.7). Davids et al. take a slightly different approach. They asked two members of a group to try to serve the ball against a wall so it bounced back to the other person. One of them did it well and the group commented that the ball toss was important. It had to be in the right place and that it was better for the person to be side on. Thus, here the emphasis was on learning from watching others and then exploring this with their own solutions. Video-recordings were made and the players could view themselves if they wished. Again the individual search for the solution was paramount.

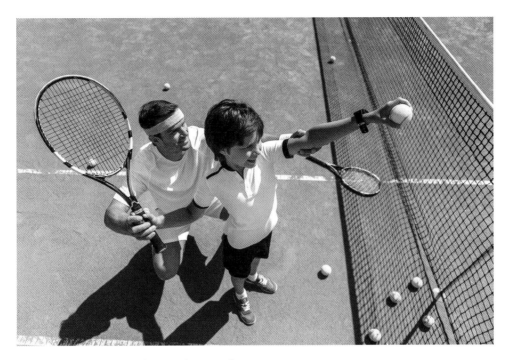

**Figure 6.7** Young boy being taught a tennis serve.

In this example, it was not just the task constraint that was being modified but the players' resources were being explored through a problem solving exercise and observation. This type of practice has great parallels with earlier ways of teaching games, such as the work of Thorpe and Bunker (1989) and the book *The Inner Game of Tennis* by Gallwey (2015), stressing relaxation and not technique solves the problem in as easy a way as possible.

In these three examples, there is no correct way to achieve the outcome. There is no criterion model, but each solution is searched for and is specific to the individual. A variety of solutions are offered by the context and the practices and learning becomes non-linear and self-organizing. The person in context is the unit of analysis with the guiding principles coming from the dynamic interaction of the child resources, the task as delivered, and the environment in which the situation is located.

## Summary

In this chapter, we have moved from the generic motor learning principles outlined in Chapter two and taken them into a situation that provides the environment and context for individual intervention. Chapter 7 will illustrate how these are put into practice with the case studies we have presented throughout the text.

The chapter covers two sets of literature concerning how present the learning situation to optimize the acquisition of skills. The first set embraces **traditional motor learning literature** that has been honed over many years. It particularly concentrates on the scheduling of practice and setting the conditions for the practice sessions. The second, coming from the **dynamical systems literature,** and emphasizes more the modification of the context and environment such that by changing the contexts, the resources of the child are constantly being modified to accommodate different scenarios. We firmly believe that these sets of guidelines complement each other and are not antagonistic as have been sometimes portrayed. Much of the motor learning literature places an emphasis on the amount, type and distribution of practice, while the more non-linear/dynamical recommendations look at the presentation and practices themselves, utilizing more contextual information.

# References

Ayres JR (1979) *Sensory Integration and the Child*. Los Angeles, CA: Western Psychological Services.

Blank R, Barnett AL, Cairney J, et al. (2019) International clinical practice recommendations on the definition, diagnosis, assessment, intervention, and psychosocial aspects of developmental coordination disorder. *Dev Med Child Neurol* 61: 242–285.

Bartlett FC (1932) *Remembering: A Study of Experimental and Social Psychology.* Cambridge: Cambridge University Press.

Bunker D and Thorpe R (1982) A Model for the Teaching of Games in Secondary Schools. *Bulletin of Physical Education* 18: 5–8.

Camden C, Wilson B, Kirby A, Sugden D, Missiuna C (2014) Best practice for management of children with developmental coordination disorder (DCD): results of a scoping review. *Child Care Health Dev* 41: 147–159.

Connolly K, Elliott J (1972) The evolution and development of hand function. In: Jones NB (ed.). *Ethological Studies of Child Behaviour*. Cambridge: Cambridge University Press, pp. 329–383.

Connolly K, Bruner J (eds) (1974). *The Development of Competence in Childhood*. London: Academic Press, pp. 15–168.

Davids K, Aradjo D, Shuttleworth R, Button C (2003) Acquiring skill in sport: a constraints led perspective. *International Journal of Computer Science in Sport*, 2: 31–39.

Davids K, Button C, Bennett S (2008) *Dynamics of Skill Acquisition: A Constraints-led Approach.* Champaign IL: Human Kinetics.

Dunford C, Rathnell S, Brannigan K (2016) Learning to ride a bike: Developing therapeutic intervention. *Children Young People and Families Occupational Therapy Journal* 20: 10–18.

Dunford C, Missiuna C, Street E, Sibert J (2005) Children's perceptions of the impact of developmental coordination disorder on activities of daily living. *Br J Occup Ther* 68: 207–214.

Fawcett AJ, Nicholson RI (1995) Persistent deficits in motor skill acquisition of children with dyslexia. *J Mot Behav* 27: 235–240.

Gallwey T (2015) *The Inner Game of Tennis: The Ultimate Guide to the Mental Side of Peak Performance*. Pan Publishers. London: Pan Macmillan.

Green PD, Whitehead J, Sugden DA (1995) Practice variability and transfer of a racket skill. *Percept Mot Skills* 81: 3, 1275–1281.

Henderson SE, Sugden D (1992) *Movement Assessment Battery for Children: Manual.* Sidcup: Psychological Corporation, p. 240.

Henderson S, Sugden D, Barnett A (2007) *Movement Assessment battery for Children 2*: Kit and Manual. London: Harcourt Assessment.

Hillier S (2007) Intervention for children with developmental coordination disorder: A systematic review. *J Allied Health Sci Prac* 5: 1–11.

Kerr R, Booth B (1978) Specific and varied practice of motor skill. *Percept Mot Skill* 46: 395–401.

Larkin D, Parker H (2002) Task-specific interventions for children with developmental coordination disorder: a systems review. In: Cermak S, Larkin D (eds). *Developmental Coordination Disorder.* Albany, NY: Delmar, pp. 234–247.

Mandich A, Polatajko H, McNab J, Miller L (2001) Treatment of children with developmental coordination disorder: what is the evidence? *Phys Occup Ther Pediatr* 20: 51–68.

Missiuna C, Pollack N, Law M (2004) *Perceived Efficacy of Goal Setting in Young Children (PEGS).* San Antonio, TX: Psychological Corporation.

Missiuna C, Pollock N, Campbell W, Levac D, Whalen S (2011) *CanChild Partnering for Change.* Hamilton ON: McMaster University.

Miyahara M, Lagisc M, Nakagawa S, Henderson SE (2016) A narrative meta-review of a series of systematic and meta-analytic reviews on the intervention outcome for children with developmental co-ordination disorder. *Child Care Health Dev* 43: 733–742.

Moher D, Liberati A, Tetzlaff J, Altman DG for the PRISMA Group (2009). Preferred reporting items for systematic reviews and meta-analyses: the PRISMA statement. *PLos Med* 6: e1000097.

Newell KM (1986) Development of coordination. In: Wade MG, Whiting HTA (eds). *Motor Development in Children: Aspects of Coordination and Control.* Dordrecht: Martinus Nijhoff, pp. 341–360.

Nicholson RI, Fawcett AJ (1999) Developmental dyslexia: the role of the cerebellum. *Dyslexia* 5: 155–177.

Pless M, Carlsson M (2000) Effects of motor skill intervention on developmental coordination disorder: a meta analysis. *Adapt Phys* Activ Q 17: 381–401.

Polatajko H, Mandich A (2004). *Enabling Occupation in Children: The Cognitive Orientation to Daily Occupational Performance (CO-OP) Approach.* Ottawa: ON: CAOT Publications ACE.

Polatajko HJ, Mandich AD, Miller LT, Macnab JJ (2001) Cognitive orientation to daily occupational performance (CO-OP): The evidence. *Phys Occup Ther Paediatr* 20: 83–106.

Polatajko HJ, Mandich AD, Missiuna, C, Miller LT, Macnab JJ, Malloy-Miller T (2001) Cognitive orientation to daily occupational performance (CO-OP): the protocol in brief. The Evidence. *Phys Occup Ther Paediatr* 20: 107–123.

Polatajko H, Macnab J, Anstett B, Malloy-Millar T, Murphy K, Noh S (1995) A clinical trial of the process oriented treatment approach for children with developmental coordination disorder. *Dev Med Child Neurol* 37: 310–319.

Preston N, Magallon S, Hill LBJ, Andrews E, Ahern SA, Mon-Williams M (2016) A systematic review of high quality randomized controlled trials investigating motor skill programmes for children with developmental coordination disorder. *Clin Rehabi* 31: 857–870.

Revie G, Larkin D (1993) Task-specific intervention with children reduces movement problems. *Adapt Phys Activ Q* 10: 29–41.

Roley SA, Jacobs R (2009) Sensory integration. In: Crepeau EB, Cohen ES Schell BAB (eds). *Willard and Spackman's Occupational Therapy*, 11th edition. Philadelphia, PA: Lippincott, Williams and Wilkins, pp. 792–817.

Schmidt RA (1975) A schema theory of discrete motor learning. *Psychol Rev* 82: 225–280.

Schmidt RA, Lee TD (2011) *Motor Control and Learning: a Behavioral Emphasis.* Champaign, IL: Human Kinetics.

Schoemaker MM, Smits-Engelsman B, Jongmans MJ (2003) Psychometric properties of the Movement Assessment Battery for Children Checklist as a screening instrument for children with developmental coordination disorder. *Br J Educ Psychol* 73: 425–441.

Shapiro DC, Schmidt RA (1982) The schema theory: recent evidence and developmental implications. In: Kelso JAS Clarke JA (eds). *The Development of Movement Control and Coordination.* New York: John Wiley and Sons, pp. 113–150.

Shea CH, Wulf G (2005) Schema theory: a critical appraisal and reevaluation. *J Mot Behav* 37: 85–101.

Shea BJ, Grimshaw JM, Wells GA, et al. (2007) Development of AMSTAR: a measurement tool to assess the methodological quality of systematic reviews. *BMC Med Res Methodol* 7: 10.

Simms K, Henderson SE, Morton J, Hulme C (1996) The remediation of clumsiness, II: is kinaesthesis the answer? *Dev Med Child Neurol* 38: 988–997.

Smits-Engelsman BCM, Blank R, Van der Kaay A-C, Mosterd-Van der Meijs, R, Polatajko HJ, Wilson PH (2013) Efficacy of interventions to improve motor performance in children with developmental coordination disorder: a combined systematic review and meta-analysis. *Dev Med Child Neurol* 55: 229–237.

Sugden DA (2007) Intervention approaches in children with developmental coordination disorder. *Dev Med Child Neurol* 49: 467–471.

Sugden DA, Dunford CD (2007) The role of theory, empiricism and experience in intervention for children with movement difficulties. *Disabil Rehabil* 29: 3–11.

Sugden DA, Henderson SE (2007) *Ecological Intervention.* London: Pearson.

Sugden DA (2006) Developmental coordination disorder as a specific learning difficulty. *Leeds Consensus Statement.* Economic and Social Research Seminar Series.

Sugden DA, Henderson SE (2007) *Ecological Intervention for Children with Movement Difficulties.* London: Pearson.

Sugden DA, Wade MG (2013) *Typical and Atypical Motor Development.* Clinics in Developmental Medicine. London: Mac Keith Press.

Thorpe, R and Bunker, D (1989) A changing focus in games education. In L Almond (Ed)., The place of physical education in schools. (pp. 42–71). London: Kogan Page.

Thelen E (1995) Motor development: a new synthesis. *Am Psychol* 50: 79–95.

Vygotsky L (1978) Interaction between learning and development. In: Gauvain M, Cole M (eds). *Readings on Development of Children.* New York: Academic Books, pp. 34–46.

Wade MG, Smith TJ (2015) Varaibility in human motor and sport performance. In: Smith TJ, Henning R, Wade MG, Fisher T (eds). *Variability in Human Performance.* Florida: CRC Press, pp. 31–50.

Wilson PH (2005) Practitioner review: approaches to assessment and treatment of children with DCD: an evaluative review. *J Child Psychol Psychiatry* 39: 829–840.

# Chapter 7

## Case studies: Support and intervention

## Support and intervention

We are presenting six case studies of children of different ages and a range of characteristics with suggestions as to what support and intervention strategies may be employed. They are not blueprints, but guidelines and suggestions gleaned from theory, empirical research and our personal professional practice that can be modified according to context, cultures and differing objectives.

The six case studies in Chapter 4 were chosen to illustrate children with a movement problem as a primary defining characteristic such as developmental coordination disorder (DCD), and those who showed movement difficulties as a secondary characteristic such as in autism spectrum disorder or attention-deficit–hyperactivity disorder. In this chapter we describe how objectives and priorities for action may be developed from the individuals' profiles.

Multiple individuals are involved in setting priorities and goals for the affected children and young people that take part in both **formal and informal** settings. Occupational therapist and physiotherapists are skilled in working with children with movement difficulties in formal settings. However, because of limited resources and their often low contact time, the challenge is for them to cascade their skills to those who see the children on a more regular basis, such as teachers and parents. We are great believers in professionals from different disciplines working together, such as in the Partnering for Change (P4C) model (see Chapter 8, page 202; Missiuna et al. 2011). In primary schools this is easier than in secondary schools because the class teacher has more daily contact with the children and can help them engage in more **informal sessions**. In addition, in both primary and secondary schools, the specialist physical education teacher is skillful in movement analysis and intervention for both high and low performers. It is our belief that much more can be obtained from these specialists so that children can be supported in context in an ecological setting.

## Developmental coordination disorder

In Chapter 4, three case studies of individuals were presented who were, or could have been diagnosed with DCD, aged 9, 13 and 20 years. Our support and intervention plans for the 9-year-old are more detailed than the other two. This is because of the developmental educational setting in which the 9-year-old is currently situated. He is in primary school that places multiple demands on the children in a range of areas and are often obligatory. We believe this child is at a stage where improvement can be optimal. Intervention here is timely, in preparation for secondary education in two years' time. The individuals aged 13 and 20, are choosing more specifically and carefully and with more certainty about the types of activities and practices they wish to be engaged in.

## Adam's summary profile

Adam is a 9-year-old boy of average ability in his school work but who has struggled with his motor skills since being a toddler, as noted by his parents and teacher, both reporting that he was clumsy. He is a slow writer and he has problems with planning and organization. He is above average in his reading skills. On the MABC-2 Checklist (Henderson et al. 2007) completed by the class teacher and parent he scored in the 8th to 10th centile range on Sections A and B. In Section C in the Checklist (Behaviours Associated with Movement Difficulties), he was scored as hesitant and forgetful and disorganized and was now starting to be upset by failure. On the MABC-2 Test (Henderson et al. 2007), he scored at the 2nd centile with particular difficulties in manual dexterity and balance. On the Detailed Assessment of Speed of Handwriting Test (DASH Barnett et al. 2010), he scored in the lowest 5% for his age group on the five tests of handwriting speed and this would be classified as slow when compared to his peers. A paediatrician noted no neurological abnormalities and the school reported no delay in his academic achievement. Unless other issues were noted, these would fulfill Criteria C and D from DSM 5 for DCD.

### *Objectives and priorities*
In his daily activities, reports attest to him having more problems on tasks that are open, with unpredictable timing and spatial demands. From discussions with Adam,

> **Box 7.1** Objectives and priorities for Adam
>
> ✓ More accomplishment in dealing with 'open' movement skills, those that are unpredictable in both timing and spatial demands, in particular ball games. This would help him play with peers.
>
> ✓ Speedier handwriting: all agreed this was a priority. The increase in speed to be accompanied by legibility. Poor manual skills also came out as a concern from the MABC-2 Test and Checklist. An improvement here would help him in the classroom.
>
> ✓ Bicycle riding: only Adam identified this as an objective, but he placed a big emphasis on it as he thought it would enable him to play with his peers.

his parents, teacher and therapist, and use of the Perceived Efficacy and Goal Setting (PEGS) (Missiuna et al. 2004) the following objectives and priorities were developed (see Box 7.1).

These were the objectives that were identified to work on in the first instance. All agreed on the first two but only Adam suggested bicycle riding. It is important that Adam's wishes are taken into account because it will motivate him to keep on task. It was also decided to try to encourage his planning and organization informally, during the directed support and intervention sessions.

## Programme for Adam

*Participation and learning*
A starting point for any programme is facilitation of **participation,** with time on task being key to any skill to be learned. Participation is linked to how the learning is organized. Many of these practices can be accomplished in school with the help of an occupational therapist or a physical education teacher assisting the class teacher. It would also be helpful if the school adopted a the P4C model (see Chapters 4 and 6).

*Translating objectives for Adam*
This large area of skills is commonplace in everyday life. They involve moving around the environment without bumping into stationary or moving persons/objects; participating in peer games, such as tag or ball skills. Most of these objectives do not have a predetermined outcome but have at their core problem-solving functional activities as the context is fluid and changeable. As we have noted, the solutions to these are temporarily organized in the neural system (often referred to as 'softly assembled' in the dynamical systems literature), to provide movement adaptations to the current challenge.

---

**Box 7.2** Open skills: examples using ball skills

Adam is particularly poor at ball games and would like to improve. A number of steps are involved both **informal and formal**. For **informal** approaches we would encourage the school to organize activities that Adam can be engaged in. This would require adapting tasks, giving a longer time for completion and making ball games easier. It would not involve formal teaching but giving Adam time on task with appropriate practice rather than him being left on the sidelines. When working in pairs or groups teachers should ensure that Adam works with empathetic who will keep him involved in a social situation. It is also helpful if one of the peers is skillful enough to 'feed' any ball to Adam in an appropriate manner so that it can be caught in an appropriately challenging manner. These school group games are important for both skill level and enhancement of social interaction.

Adam chose **tennis** as the game he wished to address, a game that can be practiced on his own, with a partner or, in a competitive situation. Tennis is an open skill and many of the variables contributing to success and participation in tennis are also the basis of other ball games, such as anticipation, prediction, control and moving to a moving object. The following tennis games and practices (see Box 7.3) can be used in more **formal settings** and they are tailored to Adam's unique profile and features. However, they are not technical and can be overseen by teacher or parent or Adam on his own. They are more specific activities rather than the informal social participation activities that take place in the course of normal daily functioning at school or at home. They are progressive in nature, moving from easy to complex and from individual, to partner and group settings.

---

**Box 7.3** Activities for tennis: part 1

✓ Let Adam choose a racket of appropriate weight, size and grip size, which should all be comfortable. (Cut down old rackets are not appropriate nor are leather grips!) He should swing the racket and hit the ball, if possible. There are now balls of different speeds (shown by colours) for different abilities and as Adam moves to a court it is advisable to move from slower balls to ones that are faster and eventually to a regular tennis ball.

✓ **On his own** to practice daily for 10 to 15 minutes. He needs a racket, a ball and a wall. The size of the racket to be geared to his size and stature.

✓ First he just bounces the ball up and down on his racket, trying to increase the number. He can do this while walking around as a progression. No instructions are given leaving him to explore all possibilities.

✓ Next, he does the same but keeps flipping racket back and forth to use both sides. A quick feedback by the instructor on grip may be helpful here. But again, exploration should dominate.

✓ Next, he bounces the ball on the floor with the racket, again noting the number of times. This is followed by walking around while bouncing the ball.

✓ Al these exercises can be modified and extended by Adam to include for example, hitting the ball in the air or letting it bounce while walking around. Technique is not emphasized, merely the outcome. If there is a marked and obvious problem in technique leading to a poor outcome, he may be asked to modify his grip, but few technique instructions should be given.

✓ A progression is to hit the ball against a wall. Start close to the wall and hit the ball directly to the wall, letting it bounce once before hitting it again. Count the number of times he can hit it as a challenge. The object is to get functional strokes that address the outcome of hitting the wall continuously. Very few instructions or feedback are provided in the first instance, leaving Adam to problem-solve himself.

✓ A starting point for any feedback is to look at his body positioning. All one needs to say is 'stay away from the ball'. This means he doesn't get too close, which automatically allows him room to swing at the ball. It also encourages the all-important movement of feet.

✓ There is no predetermined outcome save repeatedly hitting the ball against the wall. Adam is exploring all of the possibilities himself and he will self-organize to discover optimum solutions. It is not simply via repetition but being flexible enough to deal with an unpredictable return of the ball off the wall. Adam will start to adjust and recognize that he is in control of this situation and alter his shots accordingly. Bring in balls of different speeds.

✓ All this can be accomplished at different distances from the wall and with an added complexity such as keeping the ball against the wall by a volley rather than letting it bounce, automatically encouraging nimble footwork that in turn provides room for an appropriate swing.

**Box 7.4** Activities for tennis: part 2

✓ As soon as possible, it is advantageous for Adam to work **with a partner/friend.** In this situation, the same practices are given except this time they take it in turn to hit the ball. This automatically brings in another variable. It is not just Adam hitting his somewhat unpredictable shot, but now he has to adjust and respond to the unpredictability of his friend, encouraging the appropriate use of feet to be in the best position to return the ball.

✓ Using cooperation also helps him learn through movement. If the return is easy for his friend, they can build up cooperation to help each other and eventually compete to try for the highest number of returns each time.

✓ **Move from wall to tennis court.** With his friend, he now moves to the local tennis court. A small group would be advantageous if this step is manageable.

✓ Start with them each other on either side of the net on the service box line, thus making it a shortened court. The net can be lowered as much as necessary, even to the floor. Again, a cooperative game involves how many times they can hit the ball to each other with one bounce.

✓ The only technique instruction given is to move the feet to provide room to strike the ball.

✓ At some time, this can be changed by lifting up the net and/or moving into a competitive game where each is trying to win a point. Again, in the shortened court, and at first in just one half of the court, i.e. either the forehand or backhand box.

✓ From these modified games they go back to helping each other by taking a step back for a few shots until they are at the baseline. This example from tennis shows how Adam can move from very simple skills to more complex ones involving a game. Variations in the context can be used making the game more complex or easy, according to progression. The only outcome is to get the ball over the net. There is no prescribed way of doing this, although some feedback is given to facilitate the problem-solving process. This is secondary to Adam discovering for himself flexible solutions to the movement problem. The context is being simplified to accommodate the changing ability of Adam and friend.

✓ A more advanced practice would be for Adam to engage in a group with a knock out game in between the service court lines. This could also involve running round to the opposite court after hitting the ball. When this gets down to last three children, the scene is pretty chaotic but enjoyable!

> **Box 7.5** Variables for Adam's tennis practices
>
> ✓ Adam is learning tennis skills in particular and ball skills in general. He is learning about moving to hit a ball using space.
>
> ✓ He is learning about an unpredictable situation and adjusting to it. Each time he hits the ball, his responses involve obtaining variability of practice and response so that he can flexibly adapt to a constantly changing moving situation.
>
> ✓ In the first instance his partner can be a friend. It could be a parent of sibling but a friend is preferable.
>
> ✓ What should their ability be? It could be one who is similar to Adam although someone better would be more appropriate as she or he could help keep a rally going and give a more consistent response.
>
> ✓ Being part of a small group performing these practices would be helpful. The next step is to mix with others in this situation. Again, choosing who to play with and when, is all-important. At the first public outing resilience will be important but his skills should be good enough to cope with playing small court tennis and from there further progressions can be made.

These can be organized into short sessions by Adam, or suggestions by friends and family. A summary of these practices is shown in Box 7.5.

Adam's tennis practice can be done during personal recreation time away from school, in school or at home with family (see Box 7.6). This type of progression can be accomplished with other open sport skills such as football, hockey, basketball, and so on, as the same principles apply.

*Options for handwriting*
Adam is 9 years of age, and although handwriting may not be a major issue now, in two years' time, he will be in secondary school and activities such as writing down

> **Box 7.6** General guidelines for Adam's practices
>
> ✓ Informal sessions built in to the fabric of daily with Adam choosing to participate when he desires.
>
> ✓ More formal short sessions on individual skills at regular intervals, 10 to15 minutes a day.
>
> • Have a friend to help after initial individual skills. Build into friendship and fun time. Enjoyment!
>
> • Concentrate on function not technique, e.g. get the ball over the net, in the goal, though the basket, or kick to a partner.
>
> • Being a problem solver with the mover constantly changing the action to meet the prevailing changing contextual demands. A never-ending flexibility of responses.
>
> • All this facilitates and encourages both participation and learning, which in turn allows more time on task, thereby improving the motor skills in this **reciprocal learning–participation transaction.**

instructions from the teacher, taking notes, copying from the blackboard will all demand an increased speed of legible handwriting.

These handwriting practices can be at school and home. In the first instance, Adam will be part of handwriting practices that are for the whole class. This is in line with the approach known as 'response to intervention' that is popular in reading. Here, the child is part of the general instruction group and, depending on how they respond, more detailed and specific practices are presented for the child to engage in.

For **participation** in handwriting, both informal and formal methods can be used at home and at school. In the first instance, it is again function and time on task we are important. Thus, if the writing is legible and speed starts to increase, technique is not mentioned. However, if there is something very simple that is obviously hindering the speed or legibility of the handwriting then the points under **learning** (see Box 7.8) should be the focus. We know that better, faster, legible handwriting is beneficial for an individual's composition. A current research project, Helping Handwriting Shine, led by a team from the University of Leeds and funded by the Education Endowment Foundation, and advice from The National Handwriting Association are helpful on this (see www. educationendowmentfoundation.org.uk for details). A partnership between home and school will enable Adam to build handwriting into daily life so that practice takes place daily. But care should be taken not to overload Adam with this. Again, activities can be split into informal and formal. We recognize this is a reductionist distinction, but it does assist in a graded approach to intervention by incorporating the chosen daily skills into Adam's life and a more formal approach to direct teaching or therapy. Similarities with Ecological Intervention and the P4C models are evident here. More informal approaches are shown in Box 7.7.

---

**Box 7.7** Everyday activities for Adam

✓ At home, he could be encouraged to keep a diary, which although not done at speed will be facilitate time on task.

✓ At home, other writing activities can be encouraged. Writing about any hobbies he has, showing people the results of his writing, encouraging this on a daily basis.

✓ At school, he could be assigned responsibility tasks in the classroom, such as drawing up lists of roles for people, helping to make posters or making logs of the days' events. All these provide more time on task.

✓ The use of different materials will also be helpful, such as paper with print of different sizes, different materials to write on, and occasionally asking him to write a little faster. Time on task with gentle encouragement to write faster will increase his speed as he becomes more proficient in the act of writing.

---

---

**Box 7.8** General activities for the learning of handwriting

- ✓ At school, the teacher can set small challenges, which are targets for Adam. When he writes, the teacher can measure the speed of his writing, place it on a chart and show him each day how is progressing. All of the writing has to be legible.
- ✓ Encouragement and praise where appropriate. Direct the praise specifically at what was being asked.
- ✓ Function is the main aim and although problem solving will take place, such as finding a comfortable posture and grip, there may be instances when instructions and feedback are necessary.
- ✓ In the first instance, look at Adam when he is writing. If the writing is slowly or illegibly then look check that
  - his chair and desk at suitable height;
  - the chair tucked in;
  - his feet are flat on floor;
  - his posture at the desk – is sitting straight to desk;
  - is he using the pencil-tripod grip, not too tight or loose;
  - his distance from the paper;
  - his use of the other hand to steady paper.

---

For **learning** handwriting, and particularly the speed, a number of activities in a more formal situation the following activities can be encouraged (see Box 7.8).

However, it is important that technical aspects such as these do not dominate the function part of the exercise, which is to produce legible writing at a reasonable speed. Function and flow with comfort are the important variables on which to concentrate (see Box 7.9).

---

**Box 7.9** Priorities for action

- ✓ Let Adam **choose the pencils/pens** from a range that is available. Ask him which he feels most comfortable with. There are now a number of options available for writing implements that are designed to suit all individuals.
- ✓ Give **few instructions about posture and paper position**. Just a couple of points unless there are big faults. No need to instruct if things look OK. Simply say, 'It's good that you are sitting in a good position so you can see the pencil and the paper. Maybe hold your pencil a little further away from the point so you can see the point'. Keep it simple; no need for detail unless there is poor posture, etc. Paper is easier if it is angled towards the child rather than flat on the table. But recall comfort and function. In addition, it may be useful to consider lined paper of various types.
- ✓ Adam can write all letters so look at families of joining letters.
- ✓ Say, 'Let's see you **write your name**. Let's see you write your name as quickly as possible, really, really quick. Now slow it down so we can all read it. Now show me your best handwriting'.
- ✓ Ask Adam to write the **first line of a diary** that he is keeping in rough; then to write it again as fast as possible. Now do one in between the two speeds and keep writing at that speed. Adam can choose these types of practice.

---

✓ Watch how he **forms the letters and words** during the writing process. Is the starting point in the correct place for the efficient and effective writing at speed? Only correct if this is hindering fast, functional, legible writing.

✓ **Planning and the organization of handwriting** can be encouraged through the responsibility of designing a simple newsletter with events that have happened during the week at school or/ and at home. A template can be given with a topic for each template and Adam has to fit the words to the template. It is giving him motivating practice in general on handwriting and this will increase his overall competence that will eventually encompass speed.

✓ Look at the **flow of the writing**. Try to ensure that there is smooth continuity in the writing, stressing the almost effortless flow.

✓ It is often a good idea to **work in pairs and small groups** where the children help and encourage each other.

✓ Use of appropriate SHINE documents when they become available (due 2020, see www. educationendowmentfoundation.org.uk for details) as well as exercises from National Handwriting Association.

✓ If Adam has a more general difficulty with manual skills, then activities involving pencil and paper on colouring, mazes, tracing, etc. and associated activities with play-dough and manipulation tasks could be introduced.

✓ Variability of practice with handwriting, copying from a book, from a white board and from dictation. Best handwriting and at speed all contribute to a class of events that will useful when Adam is presented with different circumstances.

Handwriting is a skill that is unlike other motor skills, such as tennis, as the outcomes are predetermined. However, there is still leeway for the individual to perform the task in his or her own way time. Variability of outcome can be seen as long as the outcome is legible and performed at an appropriate speed.

*Bicycle riding*

This activity is totally different to handwriting and ball skills, not only because it is a gross motor balance skill, but also because of the environmental circumstances in which the child is moving. It involves total body movement, often within a moving environment, with moving objects and other people. There is the additional factor of safety that must be taken into consideration. Thus, the usual way to teach cycling is to use a system that breaks the skill down into a number of component parts. There are a number of websites and booklets on this and the following is a summary of some of the approaches used (see Box 7.10). Good sources and references for this include the work done by Carolyn Dunford and colleagues (2016) at Brunel University and Anna Barnett and colleagues (2011) at Oxford Brookes University. (A real-life example is provided by Anna Barnett in Chapter 8.)

Although Adam is to be encouraged to find his own solutions to the balance issues involved in bicycle riding, safety is the overriding concern.

---

**Box 7.10** Progression of bicycle riding practices

✓ It is probably better to wear long trousers and shirts with long sleeves, although care should be taken with the chain and long trousers.

✓ Off-road practice to start, such as in playground, with no traffic.

✓ Bicycle should be appropriate to child's size and wider tyres are better.

✓ Ensure child is not tired, i.e. not after a long day at school, unless really motivated. Weekends and holidays are good.

✓ First practice step is to have the child walk the bicycle and stop and start using brakes to command.

✓ Follow this by asking the child to walk and steer the bicycle in and out of cones with supporter walking along the side.

✓ Drop the saddle so that the child's feet can rest flat on the ground.

✓ Remove the pedals so the child can 'scoot' with the bicycle.

✓ With pedals off, child scoots and stops and starts according to commands.

✓ Still scooting, the child steers in and out of cones and obeys stop and start commands.

✓ Scooting and coasting for longer periods of time and distance.

✓ Pedals back on and riding with full support, stopping and starting on request. Support can be seat or harness, with supporter walking/running alongside, holding the saddle from behind allowing supporter to let go without child knowing when.

✓ If stabilizers are used, raise them gradually.

✓ A gradual reduction in support and activities as above, such as weaving in and out of cones, etc.

✓ This eventually leading to cycling with supervision in more complex environments, such as on side streets and roads.

✓ Overall, a graded set of practices increasing in demands according to the child's progress.

---

Again, function is most important with modification of the context and implements being the important variables rather than the technique.

The three activities of **tennis, handwriting and bicycle riding** require different approaches. Handwriting is contextual and the whole product is introduced at the start; only if there is difficulty in forming letters would we advocate single letter training. At this age we would advocate writing whole words and sentences that are appropriate to the child's life. We prefer this approach to breaking the task down into its component parts, such as cycloids, etc. In Adam's case, he can write all the letters and he can write legibly, but he is slow and so we are presenting activities that first enable participation and secondly help him write faster.

The cycling and tennis regimes are different. Adam cannot perform the whole task in either and so they must be simplified into their component parts. The idea here is to make sure that all the parts move seamlessly into one another with functional modifications of the context. There is minimal overlap of the parts, but the gap between the tasks should not be so great as to create unnecessary redundancy. All the tasks need to be motivating in their own right.

Adam is a bright boy and all the practices for the activities can be explained to him so that he is totally aware of what is happening. He had a couple of other objectives that involved planning and organization. These are both part of a *moving to learn* group of activities and could be readily incorporated into the *learning to move activities* described above.

*Strategies*
As well as the above points, there are some general points that will make the activities easier for Adam. **For tennis, bicycle riding and handwriting it is better to modify and adapt the context and task as much as possible to make the task simpler** and increase the possibility of participation leading to learning. Changing the environment is much easier than changing Adam, and by doing the former, the latter will follow suit and so this cycle of change and improvement will continue. In tennis, make the court smaller, use slower balls; and easier rules to facilitate engagement. In handwriting ensure the writing implement is as comfortable as possible, the paper and posture appropriate and the material to write about interesting and motivating. For bicycle riding, it is crucial that the bicycle is suitably adjusted in terms of size and type and there are graded practices.

Our teaching and coaching here still follows our basic principles of function being the primary outcome. It may differ in the three activities but function over form is our emphasis. In handwriting, there will be more emphasis on technique as a peculiar technique may be restricting both speed and legibility, but within these constraints the child is free to choose their own way; it is still a problem-solving activity for them. For both bicycle riding and tennis, the outcome is all-important, and technique is introduced only when it severely hampers outcome.

# Jenny's summary profile

Jenny is a 12-year-old girl, highly intelligent, quiet and reserved, who has had a history of what could be called neuromotor difficulties. Her birth was normal at term (weight of 2.5kg), but with delay in all her motor skills. In her first year of life she was assessed for suspected cerebral palsy (CP) because of hyper tonicity in her arms but this disappeared, and no diagnosis of CP was ever given. She has an articulation difficulty and has had speech therapy over the years. She is an extremely high achiever at school. She is 'clumsy' but is a neat but slow writer; she does not text in public. She is beginning to have difficulties socializing, although she has two close friends who support her. She is articulate and honest and would like help.

Jenny scored in lowest 1% in both the MABC-2 Checklist and Test (Henderson et al. 2007). On the MABC-2 Checklist Jenny scored low in Sections A and B, indicating that her difficulties were in manual skills, whether manipulation or reaching and grasping and intercepting and in gross motor skills in Section B involving a moving environment. In Section C, Behaviours Associated with Movement, she has difficulty in planning and organization, but her self-concept is still OK. She is not overly upset by failure and has a strong motivation to succeed.

*Objectives and priorities*
From discussions with Jenny, her parents, teachers and therapist the following objectives and priorities were developed (see Box 7.11).

Jenny has a number of positive characteristics that will be helpful for any intervention (see Box 7.12).

**Box 7.11** Objectives and priorities for Jenny

✓ Work on manual and fine motor skills, such as writing, general keyboard skills and texting, with help from her two close friends.
✓ Communication, in terms of articulation and general socializing. Continue with speech therapy, but ask therapist to cascade practices to Jenny's parents, teachers and friends. Use of two close friends to help her extend friendships and through these participate more in movement activities.
✓ Use of 'easy' gross motor activities to help Jenny gain confidence and encourage more participation in everyday tasks.

**Box 7.12** Positive aspects that will help Jenny

✓ She is bright and motivated, making it much easier to devise practices for her.
✓ She has two friends who are keen to help her. Jenny's views are paramount here and she has articulated them with clarity, precision and certainty. She wishes to improve her manual skills from handwriting to keyboard and texting skills and manipulation of small objects.
✓ To participate in manual skills, she can be proactive in a 'safe' environment with her two friends giving her confidence for when she has to perform in a more public manner.
✓ She would wish to improve her gross motor skills so that she can interact socially with others in a more comprehensive manner.
✓ For her second objective of improving gross motor skills, again the use of her two friends is all-important. Sympathetic, helpful friends and how can contribute in a massive way to Jenny's outcomes. This is not only true of children with movement difficulties but also in other areas of developmental disorders, such as autism and attention-deficit disorder. It is particularly important in early adolescence when peers are so important in the individual's life.

## Programme for Jenny

### Participation and learning

As both manual and gross motor skills are being identified, a general programme of intervention should be devised. Our view is that any support given by the two friends is paramount and that parents and teachers are kept in the background for the time being. They can be supportive in several ways, but formal intervention practices are not yet needed.

Translating objectives (see Boxes 7.13–7.16).

Again, Jenny's friends can assist here and the actions on texting can be extended to the keyboard. They can play games together, extend messages, sending each other interests they have in common.

Although she has some motor skills difficulties, Jenny has a number of positives. She is bright, understands the situation, and is highly motivated. With help, she will choose the appropriate activities and with the two supportive friends will increase the all-important

---

**Box 7.13** Manual skills

✓ For the manual skills, short fast games can be included.

✓ Texting between the friends, sending funny messages, jokes, when they are all together in the same room so they can interact and joke with each other. No instructions are given, just encouragement to participate.

✓ Friends can show her the short cuts there are on the phone for texting. There is no need for formal lessons or instructions on this, as her friends will have a better idea of what to do with their phones than most teachers or adults. Function in a social setting is the priority.

✓ She is practicing what her two friends are showing: watching them and learning from them in a context that is mutually enjoyable for all.

✓ All of this is functional yet unpredictable, with the actions developing from texts as they progress.

---

**Box 7.14** Keyboard skills

These may require more formal instruction from the teacher and short, sharp practices for Jenny to practice on her own.

✓ They would include where to place fingers on the keyboard. A decision to be made here is whether to teach the full-finger approach or to restrict it to the first two fingers on each hand.

✓ Using two fingers on each hand will give a faster start but will be more restrictive later. This should be Jenny's choice guided by the teacher.

✓ There are a number of commercial products for pupils that are fun and fast ways to improve typing and other keyboard skills; such games as can be used by Jenny on her own under the guidance of the teacher and or parent.

---

**Box 7.15** Handwriting skills

*These can be improved by age-appropriate extensions of the programme for Adam. Jenny has good handwriting and is coping, but she is slow.*

- ✓ More practice at speed is a way forward, keeping a diary and writing quickly in it will encourage this
- ✓ Variability of practice with speed emphasized, then 'best' handwriting and then following instructions given in different modalities from a white board, aurally by teacher, or copying from a book as well as free writing.
- ✓ As she is very bright, she could be encouraged to write short stories, again at speed, checking legibility as she goes along.
- ✓ She is self-motivated and can do these in her own time and place. No instruction to be given except if there are obvious technical issues that are slowing her down.
- ✓ General manual skills such as manipulation would give Jenny a broader base from which to practice her keyboarding and handwriting.

---

**Box 7.16** Gross motor skills

- ✓ Use of friends so important again here. At 12 years of age Jenny is not going to be motivated to do the practices that one gives to 6- to 9-year-olds. Again, we would encourage the inclusion of the two friends to help build activities, as much as possible, into her ordinary daily life routine.
- ✓ In talking with pupils of Jenny's age we have been informed that they occasionally do a lot of running and chasing and sometimes play tag at break time. But they are not primary motor activities; social activities such as talking with each other predominate. These activities would encourage Jenny in the all-important area of making good friends, which can lead to other benefits later. These are to be encouraged as much as possible with sympathetic friends.
- ✓ Dancing is one activity that often appeals to both sexes at this age and can be performed in private and/or with the two close supportive friends. Dancing to the music they choose in a small group encourages time on task and may eventually lead to dancing in a more open situation with others involved.
- ✓ Other gross motor activities may include cycling and 5(or less)-a-side ball games. However, Jenny's choices are paramount.

---

participation rates in her recreational and school activities, leading to an increase in functional daily skills.

## James' summary profile

James is 20 years of age and in his first year at university studying chemistry. He has a history of movement difficulties and had a diagnosis of DCD at 9 years of age. This diagnosis fulfilled all of the criteria from DSM IV-TR (APA 2002), which was the prevailing criteria at the time.

When tested in childhood on the Movement ABC-1 Test and Checklist, scores from both parents placed him in the typical range on practically all areas of fine motor demands. Overall, he was in the 5th to 15th centile, which would be in the range for monitoring rather than immediate action. However, the occupational therapist thought that his skills in the moving environment and balance and recreational skills were poor enough for her to recommend that Criteria A and B of DSM-IV were satisfied. On an IQ test he scored 136 with little discrepancy between verbal and performance scores. He was given a diagnosis of DCD. He was distressed about his poor motor skills, although he ran in the school cross-country team and enjoyed this activity gave him a social context. But he could not ride a bicycle and did not learn to drive, two activities that he believed restricted his social life. He would like some guidance and support and moving to university may help this.

### Objectives and priorities

Following discussions with James and advice from the University Diversity Officer, the following objectives and priorities were developed (see Box 7.17).

James identified both of these as aims.

Currently, it is not thought that driving is a priority for two reasons. First, at University a car is not a necessity as he lives in a university hall of residence half a mile from campus. Secondly, learning how to ride a bicycle may help those abilities such as moving in a moving environment that will be necessary in the future when he does start to learn to drive.

### Participation and learning

#### Translating objectives for James

We know from recent research, much of it conducted by Kirby et al. (2008a, 2008b), that both motor and non-motor variables are important in the life of young adults. Indeed, the non-motor areas often make up a significant part of the individual's life. The motor

---

**Box 7.17** Objectives and priorities for James

✔ Some tailored programmes supported by friends may be the way forward. Joining recreational clubs at University may help James to interact socially with others and could include various fitness classes involving coordination activities, not so much for the fitness but helping with coordination and friendships. This is a new environment and he can make a fresh start in this new context.

✔ Riding a bicycle was the first thing that James mentioned and said that if this could be accomplished it would change his life substantially. This will take some care and attention as James has most difficulties when moving in a moving environment.

activities that are crucial in a young child's life such as dressing and manual skills have usually either been overcome by the time she or he reaches adulthood or, at least, compensated by other activities. However, the consequent effect of the motor activities can be seen in other areas such as socializing, recreational, leisure activities and mental health.

*Join a club*

In all our recommendations for James the first priority are his wishes and goals, although advice from various quarters can be obtained if he so desires. There will be a Student Disability Service or equivalent at his university and he may choose to contact them.

With this in mind, we would recommend that the first action James takes is to **join a club** (see Box 7.18) that will take care of his obvious running and other cardiovascular skills. This can be a cross-country group or a walking group. This will achieve a number of objectives.

If James feels his first priority is to continue with his running, then such a club would take priority. Many university running clubs have graded groups so that James would be able to find one that suits his ability and his personality. If he is a little nervous, he may choose a group that is slightly below his ability so that he can fit in more easily in the first instance. He then could move up to a group of higher performers.

Walking groups are always social and, depending on which university he attends, there will always be countryside to walk in that is both interesting and challenging. These groups usually walk once a week with occasional weekends away. Again, this is a good way to meet new people and socialize as well as maintaining basic fitness.

There are new demands at university, with support being less available than in previous times of his life. Parents are not around and so it is imperative that James has some friendship groups. He has a number of skills to offer. He is obviously bright enough and has a pleasant disposition and so he needs to place himself in situations where like-minded students are present. Joining one of these clubs will

---

**Box 7.18** Issues to consider

- ✓ First, he will be able to meet new people in an environment in which he has shown himself to be capable. In Chapter 8 Amanda Kirby points out that growing up with DCD often restricts friendships and interests and in James case this is true. Thus, meeting new people in an environment in which he is comfortable is the first step to progress in other areas.
- ✓ This step is important because as the individual reaches adulthood the lines of support reduce and the scaffolding that is present in the earlier life is not as readily available.
- ✓ Support and resources are fewer whereas expectations in adulthood are higher.
- ✓ The individual must take some responsibility and for James to join clubs is an important first step in this regard.

---

**Box 7.19** Benefits of James' objectives

✓ He is taking responsibility for his own future in the short- to medium-term.

✓ This may evolve into more life-changing actions both at university and beyond.

✓ He will become fitter by his regular activity, leading to an overall healthier lifestyle.

✓ His representative activities will boost his ability in such as areas as planning and organization.

✓ This fitness together with his new contacts will boost his self-concept.

✓ This increase in self-concept will help him socialize in more and in better ways.

✓ He will gain new friends.

---

help. In addition, he may wish to have a position of responsibility such as a 1st year representative, or other such role, which will keep him in regular contact with others in that particular group.

This overall positive action on James's part has a number of benefits (see Box 7.19).

*Bicycle riding*
Because he is much older, the bicycle-riding programme we set up for Adam earlier in the chapter will need to be modified for James. There are, however, some similarities and it is these we present together with comments about a programme tailored specifically for James (see Box 7.20).

---

**Box 7.20** Bicycle riding activities for James

✓ Off road practice to start, such as in playground or other similar space with no traffic.

✓ We would recommend a hybrid bicycle or a mountain bicycle, both easier and safer than a road bicycle, which has narrower wheels and tires. If he is to use it for commuting, then the hybrid type is better, if more off road then a mountain bicycle is preferable. Our guess is that a hybrid bicycle with straight handlebars and city-ready is the one that will be most appropriate and multi-purpose. There will be room for a fitting for panier bags if required. Ensure bicycle is good fit.

✓ Walking with bicycle and getting on and off bicycle.

✓ Walking bicycle in and out of cones.

✓ Getting on bicycle and free-wheeling down a slope to command.

✓ Pedalling bicycle with supporter holding saddle.

✓ With a friend, ride on country roads with little traffic to practice balance.

✓ With a friend, move to an urban road with little traffic but signals and stops signs.

✓ Gradually increase complexity of urban cycling.

✓ Riding to university from accommodation with a friend is always beneficial.

---

Adults with movement difficulties, like James, are being identified more regularly. It is important that he chooses his own goals. Equally important are the careful, but non-intrusive, support systems. There is no prescribed way of doing this, being unpredictable and always James' choice. As with the other individuals, function dominates over technique, which only becomes necessary when poor technique interferes with function.

## Children with other developmental disorders

The following case examples are of children who have a primary developmental condition, but also have movement difficulties as a secondary characteristic.

### Marie's summary profile

Marie is a 12-year-old girl just starting the first year of secondary school and has been diagnosed with attention-deficit–hyperactivity disorder (ADHD), primarily because of her attention difficulties rather than hyperactivity, although she does occasionally show signs of impulsivity. The diagnosis of ADHD was given according to the DSM-5 (APA-13) criteria evidencing more than six of the characteristics listed in the DSM-IV diagnostic criteria. Her parents and her teachers were given the Connors' Checklist to complete and scored her low on attention, with some associated learning difficulties Other issues included low scores on executive function, mainly identified by the parents.

In class, she scored around the 15th to the 20th centile in most subjects but had no extra support. As she developed, problems started to appear more at home. Her gross motor skills have been poor throughout her childhood; thus, participation is a major issue with lack of attention thought to be the primary cause. She cannot ride a bicycle, her fine motor skills are poor and she is slow to dress in the mornings, often missing the school bus.

 Her low self-concept is not helped by her poor motor performance. All agree that she needs to participate more as an aid to overcoming some of her attention difficulties, by incorporating **Moving to Learn and Learning to Move** activities. She has not had a formal assessment of her motor skills but she and her friends and family believe she is a classic case of **moving in order to learn other attributes**.

## Programme for Marie

In discussion with Marie, her parents, teachers and others, it was agreed that her attention was the priority to work on and a programme of learning through moving involving attention skills, together with increasing her participation rate was the best approach (Boxes 7.21–7.27).

---

**Box 7.21** Translating activities for Marie

✓ Enhance her attention skills through a variety of methods.

✓ Facilitation of participation in movement situations as a way forward will help both her motor and her attention skills. To facilitate participation, the context/environment will need to be more accommodating to her needs.

✓ Marie may choose which tasks she would prefer to learn, such as dressing quickly, texting, or any other skill that she feels she really needs.

✓ Provide her with motor activities that are achievable reasonably quickly but need a little attention before she can gain success. This will not only aid her attention but also give her much needed confidence and heighten her self-esteem.

✓ Tasks that involve planning may help her executive function capabilities.

✓ The ideal scenario for these motor activities should involve one or two close friends who have empathy with her difficulties and are willing to help.

✓ Engage in specialist training sessions that concentrate, slowly, on gaining attention through movement.

---

**Box 7.22** Attention enhancing activities

Enhancing her attention skills may encourage and give her confidence to participate more. The concept of attention is not unitary and can be broken down in various ways. We prefer to break down the concept as follows:

✓ **Coming to attention:** activities to gain Marie's attention in the first instance.

✓ **Selective attention:** activities that help Marie concentrate on the appropriate part of any activity.

✓ **Sustaining attention:** activities that help Marie stay on task for a longer period of time, possibly measuring this and providing encouraging feedback.

✓ **Freedom from distraction:** coupled with sustaining attention, activities that provide constant interest in themselves so that she has no need to look elsewhere for interest. Not easily distracted

✓ **Control of impulsivity:** activities that ask her to first look, listen and think before acting.

---

There are activities that can be given, some of them overlapping, that can help Marie with attention and impulsivity. When devising a programme of support we would target these as a priority, embedded in movement skill activities that Marie enjoys, and indeed chooses. Marie does not have much difficulty with impulsivity, but her problems are with attention. In any set of guidelines there are a number of principles that will apply. Box 7.23 shows some that may be helpful.

We are emphasizing that Marie has needs in the movement domain and these are not helped by her occasional impulsivity. Thus, in order to participate in improving her manual skill she can practice in a 'safe' environment with her friends, giving her confidence for when she has to perform them in public.

**Box 7.23** Strategies for Marie

✓ Any activity should be interesting and motivating to the child. It is always better if they are Marie's choice (see below), but she may have to engage in some of your choices to accomplish the objectives of the activities. If Marie is reluctant to do that let her choose hers first on condition that she does yours next.

✓ Rewards are good but need to be earned.

✓ Small tangible rewards can be stickers that she can exchange for things she likes to do; they should always be accompanied by praise.

✓ Move as quickly as possible from tangibles to praise on its own.

✓ Praise is for the job done, not just the person. Not just, 'Well done You are a good girl' but 'Well done Marie, you have done exactly what we asked'; or 'Well done, you stuck at it and look how well it has turned out'; or 'See how well you finish the task when you pay attention'.

✓ Eventually get to a stage where you can ask 'Why do you think you did well on that task?'

✓ Get to the point where she can attribute her success to 'sticking' at it (i.e. sustained attention) not that it was *easy* or she was *lucky*.

✓ If you do manage to get some 'sessions' with her it is better that they are 'little and often' rather than long and infrequent. Ten to 20 minutes gradually increasing in time and/or complexity say four to six times a week is better than 1 hour once a week. Think of your own piano practice!

✓ Stress control of the activity all the time, not speed. How slowly, how neatly becomes the end target, not how fast.

✓ You may wish to use words like 'Marie when we play at this I want you to STOP–LOOK–THINK before you do anything' keep stressing this.

✓ You may also wish to ask 'What do you think this task is asking you to do'. We are trying to get Marie to think about the task and start to control her own learning and not just do follow your instructions. It can then merge into some really good questioning that can scaffold her learning.

✓ There is a highly recommended form of questioning (The Zone of Proximal Development) originated by a Russian psychologist Vygotsky. It is the result of an assisted form of questioning and it means that Marie on her own can reach a certain level of achievement, but with 'scaffolding or assisted questioning' can achieve much more. The individual cannot go straight to the answer but with carefully structured questions that she can answer, she actually discovers the answer for herself. It takes skill and time but encourages the child to SLOW DOWN AND THINK!

✓ The aim of the strategy is to get Marie to slow down and take control of her own learning. This will not happen overnight as she is young, but it will help her impulse control.

It is recommended that the activities are attempting to address both these needs. In some activities there is a greater emphasis on the control of impulse and on others the emphasis is on the motor control. Getting the balance right involves skillful 'teaching' and good observation.

### Prolonging activities for Marie

This is simply asking her to perform a movement for a longer duration. This may then transfer to other activities. The choice of activity is crucial as she may choose one that

**Box 7.24** Slow-fast-normal paced activities for Marie

✓ Marie may have to perform activities at a fast, slow, or normal pace. Thus, the following activities may be of use.

✓ Walk a marked out curved path, about 10m in length.

✓ Roll a large ball along the path.

✓ Ride a tricycle along the path.

✓ Draw a line like the path on the paper; this can be traced or drawn between lines.

✓ 'Walking' crayons down the page.

✓ Winding in a fishing reel, maybe 3m or so.

✓ You can ask her to perform these activities at a fast, then slow, then normal speed, each time encouraging her to pay attention by looking at what she is doing and not drifting off. You can take lots of measurements to show her how fast or how slowly she performs the activity or the **difference between her fastest and slowest speed.** What is her **normal** speed? By engaging them both together she will be acquiring both impulse control and motor control.

**Box 7.25** Relaxation training for Marie

✓ These activities may help her consciously relax. She may not know why she is doing the actions but just 'does them'.

✓ Lie down on a mat on back with knees slightly bent, may be with a roll underneath them to make it comfortable and a small pillow under the head.

✓ Ask her to tighten and then relax various parts of the body: 'So Marie, can you make your body stiff like a piece of wood/metal; now can you make it like jelly?' 'Can you make just your arm stiff, now like jelly?' 'Can you make one stiff and one like jelly?' These activities are not easy but it's good to try to alternate the stiff-relax-stiff-relax modes. The idea is to get her to know more about what her body is doing. Often a lack of awareness of this is a cause of impulsivity.

✓ Try to get her to relax and tighten her jaw and face muscles, which are often a source of tension.

✓ Other instructions may include 'Can you make your body be heavy/light?' 'Can you make your body sink into the mat?' 'Can you make it float?'

✓ Ask her to touch her right leg with her left arm (and vice versa); if she does not know her left and right yet, show her.

she wants to do all of the time so you have to move her on to tasks that are less her preference but important in her daily life (see Box 7.26).

Activities selected by Marie and her friends can help. They can be performed in both formal and informal sessions at school, at home, with friends, or on her own. Many of them address more than one of the objectives listed earlier. Her challenges have been with attention, leading to other difficulties, movement skills being one of them. By using attention activities she is learning through movement, with the aim that these will transfer to other aspects of her life. As with all programmes, close monitoring of the situation is essential to ensure that progress is optimal.

---

**Box 7.26** Prolonging activities for Marie

- ✓ Walking lines of increasing length in a 'normal' controlled manner is an obvious activity.
- ✓ Another activity that is good but may be difficult for her is to place a tennis ball on a square piece of wood (about 15 to 18 square feet or diameter) and ask her to walk around while keeping the ball on the board.
- ✓ Drawing in between lines on paper with the track increasing in difficulty and complexity will help her with her drawing.
- ✓ Changing the complexity or difficulty of any task is an essential part of any support system. She needs challenging at her level or just above; too easy and she does not progress; too difficult and she gives up.

---

**Box 7.27** Impulse control activities for Marie

- ✓ These have to be done less frequently than the attention activities.
- ✓ They involve asking her to show how slowly she can move, e.g. walking as slowly as possible on a line.
- ✓ How slowly can she get up from lying down or sitting down with crossed legs?
- ✓ Use of white/blackboard with 'tracks' on it, how slowly can she 'drive' the car through on the 'road'?
- ✓ Slow music being played as she does these activities may help.

## Andrew's summary profile

Andrew is a 9-year-old boy who has been diagnosed at age 5 years with high functioning autism (originally Asperger syndrome under DSM-IV (APA 1992); but generic autism spectrum disorder (ASD) under DSM-5 criteria. This led to him being disadvantaged in social and school settings. Observations that gave rise to concern started when Andrew was a 2-year-old toddler and eye contact was lacking. At 3 to 4 years, he lacked the appropriate use of language and other forms of communication such hugging and touching. At 5 to 6 years his speech was syntactically good but the context in which it was used being highly inappropriate with language usually one-sided and self-referenced. He engaged in simple stereotypical behaviours and was reluctant to change. His parents have been excellent in understanding these behaviours and have attempted to accommodate them. At preschool, these were also accommodated in a pleasing manner. He has maintained a good level of achievement but still exhibits socially inappropriate behaviours.

He also has motor difficulties, which may seem relatively minor by comparison to his other needs, but they are real and unfortunately are now becoming a source of stress for him. His classmates are now less tolerant of his behaviours. This, combined with his clumsiness (he cannot ride a bicycle and has an awkward running style), has caused him to become the object of ridicule. He is quite isolated both in school and outside of school where he has difficulty making friends. However, he does have two fellow pupils, who live near his home, and although not close friends, they do offer support. He is also learning to swim, and the friends have offered support in this area.

When Andrew discusses his condition, he does it mostly from his viewpoint but does recognize that others may be able to help him. His parents and teachers feel a new approach is required to help him cope when he moves up to the much bigger and probably threatening world secondary school in 2 years' time.

Most of the objectives and priorities for Andrew come under the rubric of **moving in order to learn.** This involves using movement as a source of motivation and context to learn through.

## Programme for Andrew

### Objectives and priorities

After discussions with Andrew, his parents and teachers the following objectives and priorities were developed and agreed. They involve social interaction as a priority and include movement activities as a facilitator of these (see Box 7.28).

With Andrew, as with many other individuals, movement activities are not only objectives in their own right, but also an aid to other accomplishments. Again, both learning to move and moving to learn are evident here, with the latter predominating.

---

**Box 7.28** Objectives and priorities for Andrew

✓ Make friends. Everyone agreed that this should be the main objective and that all other objectives could feed into this. There is strong evidence that individuals with ASD cope much better if they have a few supportive friends who understand and have empathy. In addition, it was thought by his teachers and parents that this objective may lead to the successful accomplishment of other objectives, such as communication and social interaction skills.

✓ Following the first objective, it would be advantageous if Andrew could be encouraged to engage more with his two 'nearly' friends in his class and then a circle of acquaintances who were part of this now trio of good friends and who understood and sympathized with his challenges. This can lead to engagement in various types of ball games.

✓ Learn to be able to swim at a level that will permit him to engage with others, possibly at a school or a recreational club.

---

### *Participation and learning*

*Translating objectives for Andrew*
Participation is all-important for Andrew and for this to occur the first step is to engage with the two friends in his class who understand his challenges and who also live nearby (see Box 7.29).

### *Circle games*
Games that involve circles are good for all children of this age. They offer planning and organizational challenges; some require ball skills and various coordination activities (see Box 7.30).

Games such as these can be extended. It is important that Andrew is an engaging and deciding participant in these games and that he becomes the person who occasionally determines what is going to happen, yet is also accepting of other's viewpoints.

These and others like them are games that have a number of objectives.

First, they will engage Andrew in social interaction and communication. It would be helpful if at least one of his friends were in the same group. It will help him engage with

> **Box 7.29** Participation and social engagement for Andrew
>
> ✓ A number of actions can be taken by both Andrew and his parents. Andrew could ask to walk to and from school with the two fellow pupils. This one may be difficult for Andrew to initiate, but a starting point would be for him to wait for them after school and ask if he could walk home with them. In the morning they could plan to call at each other's houses at a set time to walk to school together.
>
> ✓ Andrew will probably need help with achieving his objectives. In their text, Ecological Intervention (Sugden and Henderson 2007) advocate the position of what they call a key person/movement coach. This would be someone who helps the young person by coordinating their support and any intervention. Thus, this person would be an advocate for Andrew, helping him plan his daily activities, calling on extra services that may help and working with the school.
>
> ✓ In Andrew's case, his parent would seem to be in an ideal situation to be his movement coach. In the first instance, the parents can help Andrew plan make the friendship of the two pupils in his class more secure. Once the walking to and from school has been established then the friendship can start to become more secure with meetings outside of these school related activities.
>
> ✓ In school, the teacher for physical education lessons can help by structuring some parts of the lesson that encourage social interaction. This would enable Andrew to engage in activities that help him cooperate and even compete with others, maintaining an appropriate social engagement such as accepting defeat or success with dignity and style!

---

**Box 7.30** Circle games for Andrew

In a circle:

- ✓ The leader demonstrates a balance activity in the middle of the circle with feet placed heel to toe, arms folded and eyes closed. Others copy and the best balancer demonstrates next the exercise, e.g. balance on one leg while catching a ball in circle.
- ✓ The leader calls out different ways of travelling around the circle perimeter: walking while straddling a line, jumping around circle, in and out of circle, moving backwards around the circle. Stop and start with music.
- ✓ All the above as a follow-my-leader game.
- ✓ Jumps in and out of circle with different types of jumps: half or full turn; one foot jump (hop) one to two feet; two to one foot.
- ✓ Ball games in circle: ball passed from person to person; roll it, bounce it; use of second ball to try and 'catch' the first ball as it moves around circle; team games for competition moving as fast as possible; use of deception: look one way pass another.
- ✓ Ball games extension: bouncing games, one and two bounces with players calling out a number to determine number of bounces. Use simple number problems to determine the number, e.g. bounce the ball 5 minus 3 times.
- ✓ Kicking ball games: ball in the centre of a circle and players pass to each other across the circle keeping the ball in the circle. Modify by player passing the ball then running to the position of the person they have passed it to.

---

others and show planning that takes account of other's needs, thus trying to establish a firmer theory of mind for him. The activities are helping him participate; he is learning through movement.

Second, these are simple coordination games that will assist in improving his coordination skills. He will be running, balancing, throwing and catching as well as doing two tasks at once, such as running and then catching and vice versa. Third, they will help his planning and organizational skills in variable speed situations. He may become flustered and then frustrated and occasionally want to drop out. The teacher/therapist should adjust to this and/or modify the game accordingly; slowing it down to a speed that Andrew can cope with and then building it back up again.

*Swimming strategies*
Andrew is not a confident or competent swimmer but he does go to the pool with his friends. This is to be strongly encouraged and could be built into a weekly routine. We recommend that his parents as well as teachers be involved in these swimming activities, with both informal water play activities and games. Box 7.31 lists several strategies available for teaching swimming.

**Box 7.31** Swimming strategies

✓ Instructions: Presume intellect but simplify language. Avoid metaphors and sarcasm. Do not rely on facial expressions to convey meaning.

✓ Allow the Andrew to utilize coping strategies including hand flapping, counting, or covering the face when over stimulated. Give one instruction at a time.

✓ Adjust the student–teacher ratio and hold classes during times when there are limited distractions. Consider a potential fear of water among older children and adult students. Relax apparel policies on goggles, caps, etc., if applicable. Some of these items may be too uncomfortable, even painful for students with heightened sensitivities.

✓ Offer an introduction to the pool environment; exposure to the noises, smells, water temperature, other activities in the pool, and lifeguards. Prepare for the loud sound of the lifeguards' whistles.

✓ Offer a 'quiet room'. This could be an area away from the noise and activities where the student could go if he needs a quiet break.

We are always keen for any activities to be life-long. Swimming is one such activity and is one that is engaged in at home, with family, and on holidays. Building Andrew's competency in water will achieve both learning to move objectives and moving in order to learn while sharing those social engagements that are a crucial part of everyday life. This activity also fits with the Andrew's other objective of becoming more social. These two will work together to make Andrew more competent and confident in his movement activities.

**Box 7.32** Swimming activities

✓ Start with dog paddle, which moves to freestyle

✓ Teach freestyle

✓ Have friend with him all of the time

✓ Try to get a feel for the water; crouch in the water; go under water for short period

✓ Blow bubbles under water, a lead-up stage to exhaling when doing swimming strokes

✓ Look at friend under water, blowing bubbles at each other, gaining confidence through friend. Push off from side of pool with friend then reach out to touch

✓ Dog paddle and reach to friend

✓ Keep tummy tucked in to float easier

✓ Try arms with head out of water with float between legs or other place

✓ Try legs with arms holding float

✓ Try both together for a short distance, three to four strokes

✓ Use flippers/fins

✓ Progressions involving water confidence as well as confidence for longer distances to swim using modified dog paddle moving to front crawl

✓ More advanced function activities such as breathing during strokes

## Paul's summary profile

Paul is a 14-year-old boy in a mainstream secondary school and is an example we often see in our schools in that he has no specified diagnosis for any condition but he underachieves in several areas. This effects his self-esteem, self-concept and friendships in and out of school. Paul's delay in motor and language skills and other forms of communication resulted in a lack of interaction with his peers in preschool. This continued throughout his primary school period. He was slow to read, is now at a level two years below his chronological age expectation; his also has problems with mathematics.

Paul has had no support for his poor motor skills, as it seems they were considered to be of a lower priority. He is keen to learn but starting to worry he will either fail or be shown to take much longer to learn than his friends. He has been tested in a number of academic and social areas and found to be, on, average round about the 15th to 20th centile in most subjects. Paul's is a common profile: no formal diagnosis of a learning difficulty or a motor difficulty, but enough symptoms to give parents, teachers and Paul himself some concern. He is aware of the difficulties and he is now at a stage where he is watching other children overtake him in most areas and his self-concept and self-esteem are suffering; he is becoming a little morose and inward looking. Motor skills can play a role here but only as part of an overall approach addressing multiple issues. Learning through some of the following movement activities may positively affect other areas of his life.

### Objectives and priorities

After discussion with Paul, his parents and his teachers, Box 7.33 shows the objectives and priorities that were agreed and developed.

## Programme for Paul

### Participation and learning

Paul is at an age where participation will lead to learning and this is best achieved in the company of friends. He has friends and is likeable and it is prudent to start with

---

**Box 7.33** Objectives and priorities for Paul

✓ Paul was very keen to develop his ball skills ability and so a programme of learning field hockey is planned (see Boxes 7.34 and 7.35). Paul thinks this is a good idea because it will involve him with others whom he knows and whom he believes will help him. His good social skills will be a real advantage here. It is also a game where he will meet new people. Starting a new skill from scratch may will introduce him to a group that does not know him well and hopefully will be welcoming.

✓ He can ride a bicycle, but he is not very confident and so an extension of a bicycle-riding scheme will be put into operation. He believes this will help his friendships.

these advantages. Open discussions with them and (appropriate) joking and banter are ways to get involved.

*Translating objectives for Paul*

Paul's school has always had a games option, but he has always followed the usual route of football or rugby. He and his friends and supporters believe that hockey may give him more confidence and skills, as well as meeting different people.

There are many programmes for learning the essential skills to participate in field hockey and the fundamentals have much in common with both tennis (see Adam's profile) and with football. Only a few practices are listed here but information on these is available on the internet so that Paul can be purposely engaged.

Much will depend upon the level of skill Paul shows and the support receives. The above practices and others are recommended for him to acquire the basics so that he can participate in practices and eventually small-side games. This will enable him to achieve the objectives of learning movement skills and also moving with others to acquire groups to socialize with.

It is more crucial for Paul to be enjoying the company of peers and being functional in a small game situation than being technical in his skills. These will come later as he uses his skills to participate more, thus completing the circle of participation and learning.

**Box 7.34** Hockey activities: part 1

On his own:
- ✓ Buy his own composite stick of correct size and weight; same criteria as for choosing a tennis racket.
- ✓ In the first instance, skilled functional stick work for Paul is a priority. Again, we are not overly concerned about technique but whether Paul has skills enough to join his peers in some form of game or practice.
- ✓ On his own with stick and ball, practice moving the ball around keeping close to stick. Games to encourage this.
- ✓ Can he 'catch' ball on stick?
- ✓ Can he tap it up and down like the tennis practice for Adam? This is hard but fun.
- ✓ Hitting the ball to a target such as a wall or fence.
- ✓ Dribbling the ball in an out of obstacles keeping it close.
- ✓ Progressions for all of these done at speed and/or in more tightly confined spaces.
- ✓ Hockey is a good sport to learn for Paul, as it is a skill that most individuals have not had much experience so the skill gap may not be as great as in other ball games.

**Box 7.34** Hockey Activities: part 2

With a friend:
- ✓ Passing a ball back and forth.
- ✓ Hitting it hard.
- ✓ Stopping a hard hit ball.
- ✓ Trying to dribble past a friend.
- ✓ Running with a friend passing ball back and forth.
- ✓ Tackling friend to rob ball.
- ✓ Hitting ball at targets.
- ✓ Within a group of four.
- ✓ Playing 'keep' for 2/3/4/5 passes.
- ✓ Reduce space in which play is held.
- ✓ Points for keeping ball, building up both cooperation and competition.
- ✓ Gradually move to small-sided games, 3v3, 4v4.
- ✓ At this stage, we would not recommend full 11v11 as in that situation the chances of Paul having much ball contact are slim. He needs as much participation as possible to acquire the necessary skills and so that he can plot his own progress on hitting, stopping the ball, tackling, accurate passing, running with the ball.

**Box 7.35** Bicycle riding

In a small group of his own age – probably 4 to 6 is a good number:
- ✓ Although Paul can ride a bicycle we feel he needs to be taken back to basics to build his confidence.
- ✓ The environment is crucially important with safety being paramount. Maybe start in a big indoor space with rubberized floor and this not being scared of falling. The complexity of the environment is then built up to being outdoors after the child has successfully adapted indoors.
- ✓ Off road practice to start such as playground or other similar space with no traffic.
- ✓ We would recommend a hybrid bicycle or a mountain bicycle, as they are easier to ride.
- ✓ Involve teams such as road safety officers where the first part of the instruction is checking the bicycle, tires, chain and learning the two activities of putting on the helmet and picking up the cycle from the floor.
- ✓ Paul is mature enough for him to take control of these important variables.
- ✓ The pedals are taken off the cycle and the saddle is lowered so he can scoot. It becomes a 'balance' bicycle, moving to one pedal on and scooting with the foot on the other side.
- ✓ Continuing with group work is preferable if Paul is OK with that as he can give and receive support.
- ✓ The stages are not rigid but geared to the progress.
- ✓ As he can ride Paul will go through the stages quickly and may often skip stages.

✓ There is no set rule save that the steps are geared to his performance. Saddle support or a T-shirt around the waist allow for support.

✓ In a safe environment, riding and steering in and out of cones and stopping and starting on command.

✓ Individuals in the group can set challenges (safely) for each other-quick stopping, turning, etc.

✓ At an appropriate time, Paul can move within a supportive small group to riding on quiet streets and then to more busy situations.

✓ It is important that these activities are done in a social situation with supportive friends. This is the mantra for all the individuals.

## Summary

This chapter describes the progression from the collection of information on the children/young people in Chapter 4 to the practical work with them as outlined in Chapters 5 and 6. Several working principles are presented that apply to all children. The first is that the set of resources the child possesses and brings to the movement situation is the starting point from which all intervention flows. All children live in a social context. The constraints of the wider environment and the way support is given affects their participation and learning. Small changes in a number of these variables will change the manner of participation and learning, and thus the competence of the child.

The information and subsequent agreement about the objectives of any programme come from multiple sources, and compromises often must be where all are comfortable with the objectives. The priorities of these objectives have multiple influences, but the overriding priority will be the views of the child.

We know that to learn, the environment has to be inviting for the child to partici-pate. This occurs at various levels. At a macro level, the social context of the child's world needs to accommodate the child and her/his needs. This will involve the home, community and school playing major roles and often having to change. Cooperation, working together and the translating of knowledge from one interested party to the other are priorities. Once the child is participating more, learning can progress and the manner in which instructions and demonstrations and feedback are given will all play a major part.

A short summary of the principles and practices used in these Case Studies is shown in Chapter 9.

# References

APA (1992) *Diagnostic and Statistical Manual of Mental Disorders,* 4th edition. Text revision. (DSM-IV). Washington, DC: American Psychiatric Association.

APA (2000) *Diagnostic and Statistical Manual of Mental Disorders,* 4th edition. Text revision. (DSM-IV-TR). Washington, DC: American Psychiatric Association.

APA (2013*) Diagnostic and Statistical Manual of Mental Disorders,* 5th edition (DSM-5). Washington, DC: American Psychiatric Association.

Connors CK, Sitarenios G, Parker JDA, Epstein JN (1998) The Revised Connors' Parent Rating Scale (CPRS-R): factor structure, reliability, and criterion validity. *J Abnorm Child Psychol* 26: 257–268.

Barnett A, Henderson SE, Scheib B, Schulz J (2007) *Detailed Assessment of Speed of Handwriting (DASH).* London: Pearson.

Barnett AL, Henderson SE, Scheib B, Schulz J (2011) Handwriting difficulties and their assessment in young adults with DCD: Extension of the DASH for 17–25 year olds. *J Adult Dev* 18: 114–121.

Dunford C, Rathnell S, Brannigan K (2016) Learning to ride a bicycle: Developing therapeutic intervention. *Children Young People and Families Occupational Therapy Journal* 20: 10–18.

Henderson SE, Sugden DA (1992) *Movement Assessment Battery for Children: Manual.* Sidcup: Psychological Corporation, p. 240.

Henderson SE, Sugden DA, Barnett A (2007*) Movement Assessment Battery for Children-2 Kit and Manual.* London: Harcourt Assessment, p. 194.

Kirby A, Sugden DA, Beveridge SE, Edwards L, Edwards R (2008a) Dyslexia and developmental coordination disorder in further and higher education. *Dyslexia* 14: 197–213.

Kirby A, Sugden DA, Beveridge SE, Edwards L (2008b) Developmental coordination disorder and adolescents and adults in further and higher education. *J Res Spec Educ Needs* 8: 120–131.

Missiuna C, Pollack N, Law M (2004) *Perceived Efficacy of Goal Setting in Young Children (PEGS).* San Antonio, TX: Psychological Corporation.

Missiuna C, Pollock N, Campbell W, Levac D, Whalen S (2011) *CanChild Partnering for Change.* Hamilton ON: McMaster University.

Pollack N, Missiuna C (2004) *Perceived Efficacy and Goal Setting.* London: Harcourt Assessment.

Sugden DA, Henderson SE (2007) *Ecological Intervention.* London: Pearson.

# Chapter 8

## Interviews with notable clinicians and academics on intervention methodologies

Anna Barnett, Reint H Geuze,
Beth Hands, Sheila E Henderson, Amanda Kirby,
Victoria McQuillan, Cheryl Missiuna,
Motohide Myahara, Helene Polatajko,
Mellissa Prunty, Bouwien Smits-Engelsman,
Marina M Schoemaker and Peter Wilson

### Setting the scene

We noted in earlier chapters that there are three types of evidence that one can use when intervening with children showing movement difficulties: **theoretical, empirical and professional endeavours**. Many of the chapters so far have included summaries of respected **empirical** work that has involved meta-analyses, systematic reviews and other summaries of research, together with important individual papers. Many of these reviews have been conducted relatively recently, such as the International Consensus Statement (Blank et al. 2019) and some meta and systematic reviews (Smits-Engelsman et al. 2013; Miyahara et al. 2016; Miyahara et al. 2017; Preston et al. 2016; Smits-Engelsman et al. 2018), which together with earlier ones (Pless and Carlsson 2000; Mandich et al. 2001; Polatajko et al. 2007; Sugden 2007; Wilson 2007; Wilson 2017) formed the basis of our empirical evidence. The chapters have also included what we believe to be relevant **theoretical** positions taken from various sources, such as the motor learning literature, child development and theoretical positions surrounding disability. In various chapters of the book we have outlined our theoretical stance, namely in an ecological standpoint, utilizing the model of child resources, environmental context, and task transactional approach (Bronfenbrenner 1979; Keogh and Sugden 1985; Newell 1986; Sugden and Henderson 2007; Sugden and Wade 2013). We are much in favour of this ecological approach to intervention, which allows various individuals to play important roles in the course of the individuals' daily activities, which results in small gains in many areas.

As stated in Chapter 6, we recognize that theory, empiricism and practice are not separate entities that overlap with each other. However, it is our way of organizing the evidence to show (1) the principles under which an approach is operating (theory), (2) the data from controlled studies (empiricism), and (3) evidence from the therapists and teachers themselves (professional practice). We believe these three make up the evidence for best practice.

In this chapter we will look at professional evidence, from respected clinicians and academics, which we believe, provide important insights into identification, through assessment and diagnosis, to support an intervention process. Relying solely on empirical and theoretical rationales, we argue, would mean that the evidence for support and intervention is lacking. Therefore, we have sought the views of these academics and clinicians on how they work and interact with children in a personal or clinical setting. We are extremely grateful for their time and expertise. The reports are left without comment but much of what they say is incorporated into the Chapter 9 'At A Glance'.

### Professor Anna Barnett

Anna Barnett is Professor of Psychology at Oxford Brookes University where her primary role has been a researcher and lecturer. She has also had other Departmental responsibilities including Head of Department and Department Research Lead. Anna has an

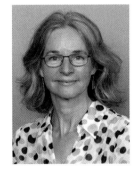

international distinguished record of research, being the author of many important papers and book chapters and being lead author of the Detailed Assessment of Speed of Handwriting (DASH) (Barnett et al. 2007) and co-author of the Movement Assessment Battery for Children (Henderson et al. 2007). She also is one of the few individuals, one of maybe two or three others, who has attended every single international conference on developmental coordination disorder (DCD) since the inauguration in London, UK in 1993 and has presented at each conference. She has also organized and hosted both UK and international DCD conferences.

In her work with families and children with DCD, she says her first step is to see how the child actually arrives at the situation (ie how a diagnosis is determined for DCD), by talking to the family, looking at the child's history in the broadest sense and then looking at motor issues the child has.

In our interview, Anna gave an account of her involvement in a community bicycle-riding course for children with movement difficulties. Bicycle riding is very often a skill that children want to learn, as it appears to be a rite of passage for many children. They want to fit in with peers, and want to participate-cycling to school or to see neighbours/relatives, family days out, school trips, on holiday with family. A core of this is participation. All want to cycle but for different reasons.

Cycling is a complex skill requiring time on task and which needs to be broken down into parts that make it less complex. The three variables (task, child and environment) are broken into a series of steps so that the learning progress is not linear but has plateaus and spurts. Anna and her team use the Task–Child–Environment model so that it is not only the deficits of the child they are analyzing, it is all three variables, such that a match can be made to the individual child. Anna stressed that each child is unique and the support and intervention is tailored to this uniqueness.

The environment is crucially important, with safety being paramount. The children start the bicycle riding in a large indoor space with a rubberized floor so that they are not scared of falling. After the child has successfully adapted to cycling indoors the complexity of the environment is built up and they are then allowed to ride outdoors.

The team works with a Road Safety Officer and the first part of her instruction is to check the bicycle, its tyres and chain and learn to put on the helmet and pick up the bicycle from the floor. This is done by all ages. Next the pedals are taken off the bicycle and the saddle is lowered so that the child can 'scoot' along. With both pedals removed the bicycle becomes a 'balance' bicycle; adding just one pedal allows the child to scoot with one foot, using just one pedal.

Some children progress very quickly and go through the stages rapidly sometimes skipping a stage, while others need more time at every stage. There is no set rule save that the steps are geared to the child's performance. All children, aged between 8 and 15 years, start at the same level in a mixed sex group with a maximum of 12 children. Group work is preferred as the children watch and support each other with praise and encouragement. The stages are not rigid but adapted to the child's progress. Eventually, the pedals are replaced and support is given as necessary by holding the saddle or the child's T-shirt while he or she attempts to ride.

It is a community-based project with the Road Safety Officer, allied health professionals (occupational and physio- therapists), disability sports officer, students and volunteer bicycle mechanics and cycling enthusiasts.

*Professor Reint H Geuze*

Reint Geuze is a distinguished emeritus Associate Professor at the University of Groningen in The Netherlands. He has expertise in developmental and neuropsychology and in neurodevelopmental disorders and has published a wide range of articles over the years on those topics. He is an expert in the field and has an enviable record on research, international presentations and publications. His primary interest is research on motor development and disorders, but he is very much aware of children's difficulties in the clinical setting. He is a keen and meticulous observer of movement, both in a clinical setting and in areas of daily living.

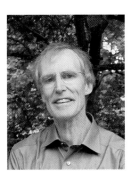

He believes that every child should have the opportunity to develop according to his or her potential. His research aims to understand the problems of children with motor deficits from basic coordination problems to related problems in daily life, and to understand individual differences.

When the children come to him for a possible guide to diagnosis, he informally interviews the parents and children to obtain details on how they cope at school and in the family, to gain an overall general impression.

Many of the parents he sees have been looking for help for their child and he makes a qualitative decision on whether they need specific clinical help or some other type of help that could be provided through parents or teachers.

If a formal diagnosis for developmental disorders is required, he recommends a consultation with the general practitioner (GP) for appropriate referral.

If they do need specific help, he discusses with the parents and the teachers what they might do to relieve the problems in carrying out activities of daily living and to stimulate motor skill development with movement games and playful exercises.

If treatment is required, he recommends functional and task-oriented treatment.

He always considers the family circumstances and so places a big emphasis on constant interaction with parents and teachers, who can encourage the child to move appropriately.

He recognizes that coordination difficulties may be due more to a lack of opportunities to develop, rather than intrinsic to the child. Again, the parents and teachers are involved in this stage, with much of it geared to finding the appropriate opportunity for the child to engage in activities to develop coordination.

He is very much interested in the co-occurring characteristics the children that may affect their daily activities and helps to clarify the priorities in how to address them.

He is prefers short, intense intervention sessions rather than long, drawn out ones and any intervention incorporates structured learning situations.

As one would expect from his background, Reint is very keen on utilizing proven motor learning principles that incorporate phases of learning, different ways of providing instructions, demonstrations and guidance, with an emphasis on feedback and how to provide it.

He is keen to point out that not every child will have a diagnosis but they all will have unique needs and that it is the ethical duty of all involved in their care to intervene and to help the child fulfil these needs.

### *Professor Beth Hands*

Beth Hands originally trained in physical Education and works at the University of Notre Dame in Western Australia. Her clinic, Adolescent Movement Programme (AMPitup) has been established for a number of years and she and her colleagues have an enviable reputation in this field. She works mainly with children and young people between the ages of 13 and 18 years who have movement difficulties. She notes that there is a need for this age group to find appropriate physical activities to meet their whole-person developmental needs. The programme is run in the University Exercise Rehabilitation Laboratory, which includes a range of exercise equipment and a hydrotherapy pool. The coaches are final year exercise science students and post-graduate physiotherapy students. The students are required to complete practical hours as part of their courses and in this way they let 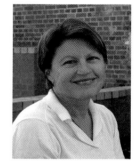 the community know that they are there to help. Because of this the community seem to be well aware of and appreciate the programme.

To be included in the programme, the young person must have a history of movement difficulties. This information is obtained by a questionnaire and talking to the parents and then confirmed by the McCarron Assessment of Neuromuscular Development (McCarron 1976).

Their overall aim is a pragmatic one: to make a difference to the daily functioning of participants and to re-engage them with enjoying physical activity. They visit the exercise laboratory twice a week for 1.5 hours, for 13 weeks in the first instance. This is the children's choice, although some have been participating in the programme for up to 6 years!

The participants work with a coach, who is supervised by an exercise physiologist, in a one-to-one situation. Although it is a clinical setting, it is also run as a research programme and so longitudinal data is collected by the students on physical fitness, physical self-perceptions, physical development and bone health.

A varied group of participants are involved, including those with DCD, mild cerebral palsy and other developmental disorders that involve movement difficulties.

The team believes it is essential for participants to engage in age-appropriate activities, often to music and in consultation with their coach about their exercise choices.

They work on pin-loaded weight machines, tapping into different muscle groups, and ergometers such as cross-trainers, rowing machines and bicycles. Floor-based exercises involving free weights, boxing, balancing and game skills are also included.

As she is trained in physical education, Beth passes on the skills of task analysis and game adaptation to the students, who modify these in an appropriate manner for the young people.

They are trained in progressions using weights and repetitions appropriate to needs and scaffolding support to assist. They do this to aid the young people to move to a community gym when they are older where the equipment may be familiar, but support may be less.

They all have individual programmes and are self-compared in progress rather than against others. They complete a perceived exertion scale after each exercise and wear heart-rate monitors so that the coaches can assess how hard they are working.

The emphasis is on positivity and success. One research project involved a 'happiness scale', completed at the beginning and end of each session. It was identified that the relationship with their coach and the exercise environment made a significant, positive impact on the participants' emotions.

They usually start the session with a warm-up on an ergometer of their choice followed by cardiovascular and strength exercises; they finish with ball games or other sport-based gross motor skills. They are taught to be sporting in both winning and losing. Each week they spend half an hour in the hydro-therapy pool.

The programme is task/skills based and founded on good motor learning principles, such as appropriate knowledge of results, clear feedback, development of aims, and how the young people rate their own perceptions of success and effort.

### Professor Sheila E Henderson

When David asked me to write something for his new book on intervention for children with movement difficulties I was hesitant, mainly because I thought I would have nothing to say that we hadn't already said together in our Ecological Intervention Manual contained within the Movement Assessment Battery for Children. Although we differ on the detail, David and I have such similar backgrounds and have worked together for so long that we share many of the ideas that we think are key to developing successful programmes of intervention for children with movement difficulties. Our common experiences can be used to illustrate just a few of these key principles.

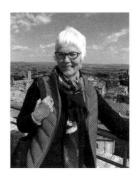

First, we both trained in the UK as physical education teachers. So, when the Beatles were singing 'All together now' and 'Yellow Submarine' in the late 1960s David and I were teaching gymnastics and games in primary and secondary schools. At the heart of our approach to teaching children, both typical and atypical, were the key concepts, *task analysis and task adaptation*. In order to put these twin concepts into practice the ability to observe movement and match the level of competence to the level of task presentation in every child in the room was crucial. With a background knowledge of anatomy, physiology and kinesiology, we were taught as students to observe movement in minute detail. This skill has stood us in good stead over the years and part of our mission to help those who work with children whose motor development is delayed has been to pass on these skills of observation.

Our Ecological Intervention Manual outlines many other principles which derive from our experience as teachers but there is one other, for which David has become rightfully (in)famous! We have all borrowed his statement that 'therapy once a week is like going on a diet on Thursday afternoon'. When we, as teachers, became familiar with the model of children with movement difficulties being offered occupational therapy once a week, we were convinced that other models of service provision were preferable. We started from the basic idea that 'little and often' is key when a new skill is to be learned, and that working one to one may not be ideal. We encouraged others to consider alternative ways of working with children with difficulties and promoted the idea of a 'movement coach' as an individual responsible for coordinating a programme of intervention, who was profession-neutral. In other words, this might be an occupational therapist or a physiotherapist, or a specialist teacher. What mattered was the availability of a responsible, committed individual with some knowledge of motor learning principles, who could take charge of a child's progress and coordinate all the strands involved. Now, the literature contains numerous examples of successful intervention programmes ranging from weekend bicycle riding programmes to intensive holiday programmes, all working with children in groups and most using non-professionals as helpers.

When we were students in the 1960s, the study of human movement as a hard science was in its infancy. Although giants such as Bernstein, Woodworth and Hughlings Jackson were working on aspects of motor control earlier in the century, much of their work was inaccessible and none of the ideas within were applied to rehabilitation for either adults or children. Slowly, however, notions such as degrees of freedom, affordances and perception-action coupling became central to the understanding of how humans (and animals) develop their truly amazing range of motor skills.

After teaching for a while, both David and I crossed the Atlantic, eager to develop our knowledge of these new developments in human movement science and to learn more about children with difficulties. This we did independently, one in the US, the other in Canada. In both cases, we were able to complete PhD theses on work relevant to our interest in children with difficulties, as well as gain practical experience in different settings. From this point on, the idea that the unit of analysis we were concerned with was not the child in isolation but the 'child in context'. So, for example, the literature on affordances led us to emphasize the importance of considering the environmental context in which the child is situated. Our understanding of perception-action coupling and degrees of freedom led to a revision of how we thought about task analysis and the manner of presentation. Together with taking account of the resources the child and his family bring to the situation, we were able to conceptualize a triad of variables that will influence the success of a programme of intervention.

On our return to the UK, we soon began to share our thoughts on how best to assess and help children whose motor development was atypical. And the rest is history: the Movement ABC Test, the Checklist and our Ecological Intervention Manual became part of one fully integrated system, designed to take the child suspected of having a motor difficulty from identification through intervention and beyond.

### Professor Amanda Kirby

Amanda Kirby is uniquely qualified to discuss the various ways she works with individuals showing movement difficulties. She is a medical doctor with great experience, who was the UK's General Practitioner of the year in 1994 and is a now Professor at the University of South Wales. She also has a PhD from the University of Leeds on young adults with DCD and associated characteristics. She has been the prime mover in many innovative approaches to children with a range of developmental disorders, with an emphasis on DCD. She set up and developed The Dyscovery Centre in South Wales, which became a beacon for the assessment and diagnosis of children with DCD and other developmental disorders. It has now merged into the University of South Wales, where she

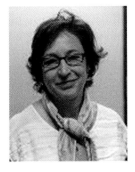

holds a chair in developmental disorders in education. She has various online initiatives such as Do-IT Profiler (http://www.doitprofiler.com), a web-based bio-psycho social assessment system. She is currently working with prisoners showing developmental disorders and learning difficulties.

Of additional relevance is that she is also the parent of a son who is now a well-adjusted, employed and very competent 33-year-old, but who in his childhood and early adulthood had difficulties with movement and other areas of functioning. Thus Amanda has a rare combination of medical, educational, clinical and parental experience.

Her current main interest is in the difficulties associated with DCD that emerging adults and adults face. She notes that for post-16-year-olds there are few support services in the UK, and if they are not being supported in education or the workplace there is a risk that they will not reach their potential. There are very few transition into adult life processes in place for these young people. She notes that what we know about the difficulties associated with DCD in adults includes the following.

First, there is a pattern of motor and non-motor challenges, both of which have an impact.

They have similarities with younger children with handwriting difficulties particularly at speed, and the need to use technology for recording.

As children, they became used to avoiding sports that needed balls skills and this often resulted in their being less fit and sometimes overweight as adults due to lack of physical activity.

Riding a bicycle has always been a challenge and as they approach adulthood learning to drive becomes a new challenge for many.

In adulthood, there are generally more choices of activities but at the same time more daily living and working responsibilities to deal with. The balance between managing work life and other aspects of their life can cause real challenges.

The non-motor, co-occurring characteristics become more of an issue in adulthood, particularly in activities such as planning and self-organization such as balancing home and work life and remembering to do routine tasks in the home.

There is also the additional impact on emotional well-being that had been noted in childhood. Anxiety can have a major impact and low self-esteem may lead the adults not to seek training or employment commensurate with their abilities.

Amanda notes that as the individual moves from childhood to adolescence and eventually adulthood, the demands and expectations go up but the scaffolding, which is support for these activities go down. Thus, a major part of supporting individuals in this phase of their life is how to manage all of these new demands. Professionals working with adults need to understand what they have come through in their lives as children and which particular route have they approached for help. Second, is the need to discover what will make a practical difference to their lives now and how shared decision making with others can help this process.

A checklist of help in this regard might include the following:

- Deciding what needs support so that the individual can function in everyday life.

- What are the priorities?

- How can the various life demands be juggled?

- What help do parents need in order to support their emerging adult offspring? So targeting parents is still a good option.

- Helping the unemployed who may be depressed/anxious because of demands that exceed their competencies.

- Try to embed organizational strategies so that they can be done automatically (e.g. use of calendars, reminders, placing objects in the same place such as keys).

- Look at sleep patterns.

- Encourage fitness and healthy eating.

- Help find a recreational interests – clubs, walking, rowing, swimming, martial arts and other skills – that are healthy but do not demand the extreme skills of ball games.

- Find a friend who is understanding and empathetic, yet pragmatic.

*Dr Victoria McQuillan*

Vicky McQuillan's interest in motor difficulties and DCD was fostered while working in child development, after having worked in orthopaedics, hand therapy and adult neurology. Initially she delivered therapy in special schools, clinics and families' homes, but later established services in mainstream schools for a growing number of children with motor difficulties and it was here she encountered DCD. She subsequently established her own occupational therapy practice and learned more about DCD from the families she met; but this raised as many questions as answers. She was particularly interested in the heterogeneity in DCD and why some children progressed while others did not. She now lectures in occupational therapy at the University of Liverpool having

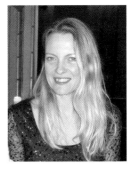

completed a PhD study focusing on the progression of children with different profiles of DCD over time.

Vicky says that the PhD was a very interesting journey in so many ways, but importantly has informed her practice. She has always been keen on detailed information gathering and taking a precise developmental, past medical and family history for each child as part of the initial assessment. A physical examination is also important looking for 'red flag' signs of undiagnosed but recognizable neurological conditions, such as cerebral palsy or Friedrich's ataxia, for example, for a differential diagnosis. However, as her understanding of the prevalence and importance of co-occurring conditions, such as ASD, ADHD and specific language impairment has grown, she is keen to thoroughly screen for conditions co-occurring with DCD and understand their impact on the child.

Through interviewing children in her own research and reading accounts of children and young people with DCD in other research, she is convinced of the importance of the active engagement of the child with DCD. Motor intervention incorporating motor learning theory also endorses active participation of the child. Occupational analysis is a core skill in occupational therapy and so a holistic analysis that includes the task and environment, alongside analysis of the child, not only aligns well with the dynamic systems approach in motor learning theory but also with occupational therapy theory. Inevitably this involves the child's own choice of activity.

Negotiating goal setting with the child and family and finding an aim that motivates and fully engages the child is crucial in intervention. However, the context of the child and family are also important, which includes their strengths, their attitude and interests and their available resources. Not least because the evidence on the detrimental effects of health inequalities and reduced participation in the uptake of health, education and leisure services is steadily growing. Therefore, she devises ways to try to ameliorate this through accessible contexts and tasks.

Intervention warrants careful consideration by all who design programmes for children with motor difficulties and DCD. She is a firm advocate of involving a number of individuals from health and educational professionals to family members who can all contribute to the intervention process. The evidence from meta-cognitive approaches and task-based approaches in an ecological setting for DCD are compelling. Handwriting, all aspects of self-care and improvement in motor coordination for function are obvious targets and desirable outcomes for intervention, and it makes sense to address these directly. However, as the engagement of all children in physical activity is low in the UK and even lower for children with DCD, it is important to help them find a sustainable and enjoyable physical activity that they can continue after therapy has finished, to help sustain the gains that they made. The physical and psychological benefits of physical activity are also well documented and so part of the therapeutic intervention must entail facilitation of community engagement in physical activity.

Strengths-based approaches to participation appeal to Vicky and despite low motor performance ability, children can really enjoy participating in physical activity and rate themselves in a positive light given the correct support, as the children in her research have shown. This must contribute to better mental health outcomes for children with motor difficulties and DCD as they grow up and a worthwhile pursuit for all those involved in their intervention.

Chloe is an example of this type of intervention. Chloe, a young teenage girl, had a diagnosis of DCD and ADHD and scored at the 5th centile on the MABC 2. Poor fine-motor control and balance were particular areas of difficulty for her, impacting on her daily functioning. She hated team sports and was reluctant to do any physical activity.

Her friends were interested in make-up and had started planning group trips to go shopping, to the school disco and the school leisure centre, but Chloe was reluctant to go. She was unable to apply makeup and was not very confident. This was lowering her self-esteem and she was starting to isolate herself. Her parents were very concerned.

Vicky first met Chloe and her parents to discuss the issues from their perspective and to establish priorities for intervention. It was important to involve Chloe in finding goals that were meaningful to her to encourage belief in her agency and to sustain her motivation throughout the intervention. In collaboration Vicky chose to tackle the difficulty with applying make-up, as Chloe and Vicky felt that this was holding Chloe back and her parents agreed.

Viewing Chloe's difficulties through the ICF framework exposes problems at three levels. She had difficulties at the body function level (her poor coordination), which impaired her activity level (unable to apply makeup), which in turn impaired her participation (joining her friends on the outings or engaging in physical activity).

Vicky decided to use a metacognitive approach, such as the Cognitive Orientation to Daily Occupational Performance (CO-OP), to help Chloe through guided discovery and use dynamic performance analysis in a realistic setting.

However, Chloe, the task and her environment all had to be considered. A stable environment for her to apply her make-up was important because of her poor balance and so a comfortable chair at the correct height for her dressing table was used, along with a mirror positioned at the correct height and angle. Three items of make-up were prioritized so as not to overwhelm her or over complicate the task; she chose mascara, eyebrow pencil and lipstick. Make-up items with large diameter shafts were selected for easy grip and an eyebrow stencil was chosen to reduce the need for accuracy.

Chloe verbalized her plan as a series of tasks within the activity, chose her makeup and started to apply it. The aim was for her to execute her plan and evaluate her own performance through guided discovery. Vicky's role was to give verbal guidance and questions for Chloe to find strategies that worked for her to improve her performance if she felt that it was breaking down. This dynamic performance analysis worked in real time and described the breakdown in order to help her understand where it happened and how to improve.

After frequent practice and targeted feedback Chloe became proficient and confident enough to join her friends. She found that she enjoyed the static bicycles and other gym equipment at the leisure centre, as they were far less demanding than team sports. She was keen to go out regularly with friends (and meet boys!). Improving her proficiency with make-up increased her self-confidence and facilitated participation in physical activity.

### Professor Cheryl Missiuna

Cheryl Missiuna is a Professor and scientist at *CanChild* at McMaster University, Canada and holds the John and Margaret Chair in Childhood Disability Research. She is an occupational therapist with graduate degrees in educational psychology and special education. She is co-developer of the Perceived Efficacy and Goal setting System and currently she is involved in Partnering for Change, which is a service run between health and education in school settings. Through *CanChild* she has produced many resources to assist those involved with children showing difficulties in movement. She has an outstanding reputation in both the clinical and research world of children with movement and other developmental disorders.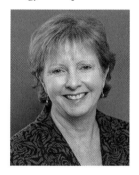

### The Partnering for Change initiative (P4C)

In many countries, such as the UK and Canada, mild motor difficulties tend to be ignored in favour of more identifiable constitutional problems, such as cerebral palsy, with finance and support going mainly to these populations. The P4C approach is a population health initiative where professionals go into schools, as a community initiative, not primarily to intervene but to find, understand and provide some support to prevent secondary consequences for children with developmental disabilities.

The P4C service delivery model has the following goals:

- To facilitate earlier identification of students with special needs.

- To build capacity of educators and parents to understand and manage children's needs.

- To improve children's ability to participate in school and at home.

- To facilitate self and family management to prevent secondary consequences.

[P4C: https://www.partneringforchange.ca/]

The P4C work involves a partnership between health and education where occupational therapists will go into schools one day a week showing a regular presence and work with teachers. The work does not necessarily involve identifying the child and working on deficits, but more in rearranging the environment and the context so the child can achieve success in a natural manner. Adjusting the size of desks and chairs, and sitting positions, are small alterations that can be made to the context without needing to give detailed instructions to the child.

P4C is about building capacity through collaboration and coaching in context.

The context is the classroom where the demands of the context are analysed for motor demand such as cutting in mathematics, and how the task can be modified to allow the child to demonstrate what they can do.

The work within P4C is very much in line with the response to intervention ideas first proposed in reading programmes. The first step is a universal programme with all children involved and the partnership includes teachers, parents and therapists and aims for success for pupils of all abilities.

For children continuing to experience difficulties differentiation takes place in the classroom and by observing the responses the partners can modify strategies and approaches for individual children.

The school stays as the context, allowing partners access to the maximum time and the maximum number of pupils.

There is no formal assessment at this stage but careful observation by an occupational therapist in partnership with the teacher is very much emphasized. In the first instance if there is difficulty, the partners will to try modify the task to ensure that the child can actually access it.

If the child continues to have difficulties another step is involved whereby families and health professionals are included to help the child. The work takes place in the school, with teachers parents and health professionals involved, and all these stakeholders learning from each other.

Early in this programme other developmental problems are looked for such as ADHD, ASD and Dyslexia.

P4C is a graded approach to intervention moving from a universal approach with all children involved through one in which some children receive extra and graded modification of the approach.

### Dr Motohide Miyahara

Motohide Miyahara has been interested in body-mind relationships, and studied relevant academic disciplines, including psychology, health education, and the art and science of human movement in Japan and the USA. After completing at PhD in Kinesiology at the University of California at Los Angeles he conducted his post-doctoral research at the University of London and the Free University of Berlin. Since taking up the academic staff position at the University of Otago, New Zealand in 1996, he has been serving as the Director of the Movement Development Clinic, a teaching and research laboratory where student teachers learn to teach and conduct case study research with children who have unique learning needs (eg, Doderer and Miyahara. 2013).

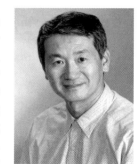

During his research and study leave in 2009 and 2015, he worked on functional magnetic resonance imaging (fMRI) research (eg, Miyahara et al. 2013) at the National Institute for Physiological Sciences in Japan. In 2017 he and his collaborators completed a Cochrane review on the task-oriented intervention effects on DCD (Miyahara et al. 2017). This has proved to be an influential document for those are interested in evidence-based intervention.

When Moto (his nickname) supervises university students who teach children at the clinic, the student teachers would start with case formulation, which is based on a cognitive behaviour approach. This involves the information from health care professionals, teachers and parents in the referral form, one intake meeting with parents and the child/pupil, and an observational assessment on the tasks to work on. He believes it is essential to listen carefully to parents and the child and prioritize specific intervention objectives. He does not feel that a single assessment (such as the MABC 2, DCDQ, or observation), worthy as they might be, automatically provides exact information for intervention tasks. He believes it is the interventionist who should interpret and translate the referral form, interview, checklist, test, and observational data into functional teaching tasks with specific progressive schedule and strategies.

The first thing that the student teacher should do is to build a rapport and relationship, which starts with the initial meeting with parents and child and followed by an intake interview.

Based on the interview, the student teacher will rank the priorities that the parents and child would. It is important to have both parties agreeing and if efforts are made to try to obtain agreement.

Moto's approach is functional task-based, that is, he looks at what the child needs in every day life. This functional-task based approach is set in the larger context of the child participating and being engaged in activities that are physically oriented.

The focus is not just on the first objective of acquiring a skill, such as tying shoelaces or riding a bicycle, but on continuing and extending participation and learning.

It is not a rigid, behavioural approach, but a more cognitive approach to achieve a change in emotions and perceptions of physical activity from a lifespan perspective, as well as the obvious improvement in movement.

He often asks the children to verbalize what they are doing, in order to obtain a fuller understanding of the whole task and its cognitive and emotional consequences.

He also looks at non-verbal cues, such as, facial expressions, gestures, and tone of voice to see if further clues can be obtained about the child's enjoyment.

When he chooses a task, he does so with a view to progressing from a single task into a bigger picture through transitional stages in life, from home, to school and to the community.

He believes the child needs a safe environment (implying that not being embarrassed in front of peers or bullied as a consequence of poor public motor performance) to learn and he sets the pace and place of the learning to the child's needs and capabilities.

Thus, overall, the programme involves a functional task-based approach using motor learning principles and then moves towards a more holistic support system, strongly encouraging participation in physical activities that eventually, may lead to more fulfilling, physical, cognitive and emotional engagement.

*Professor Helene Polatajko*
Helene Polatajko is researcher, educator and clinician. Her clinical experience is primarily in the area of paediatrics, most especially with children with DCD or other learning-based performance problems. Her research has been focused on intervention and outcome measurement. Her particular interest is in exploring how cognitive strategy use can support skill acquisition among individuals with performance deficits. She is Professor in the Rehabilitation Sciences Institute and the University of Toronto Neuroscience Program and Professor and Former Chair of the Department of Occupational Science and Occupational Therapy at the University of Toronto. Dr Polatajko has held grants in excessive of $10,000,000, and has a publication record of over 200 items including books, book chapters and peer-reviewed articles. She has given over 500 public lectures around the world including conference presentations, invited talks and keynotes. Recently she gave a TED for TEDxToronto talk on the topic of strategy use and skill acquisition. She has received numerous national and international honors and awards. Her work on

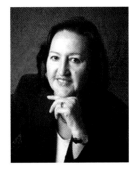

Cognitive Orientation to Daily Occupational Performance (CO-OP) is known and followed world-wide and has received critical acclaim from academia and clinical settings.

Helene illustrates her views by talking about a recent conversation she had with the concerned mother ('Jane') of a 6-year-old boy ('Bobby') who was experiencing severe performance problems and had been given a diagnosis of developmental dyspraxia. She started by asking the mother to describe the child's performance: what the child can and cannot do well; what he does and does not do, and, what things he cannot do well, but wants to do.

Her aim was to find out where the problem lay? Is it in knowing what to do, how to do it, or being able to do it? For example, if he is poor at buttoning his shirt, writing or riding a bicycle, does he have an idea about how to approach these tasks? How general were any deficits or were they related to some specific issues? In Bobby's case he had good problem-solving strategies for certain things but not for others. For example he had no idea how he might start to button his shirt or write, so he avoided doing most things that required motor skills that were new for him. Helene then asked Jane if Bobby realized that he was good at problem solving? The idea was that this ability could be harnessed to help solve his performance problems. A major interest for Helene is understanding the problem-solving abilities of children and their appreciation for that ability. Are they good or poor at this in general, or are their abilities specific, and importantly, do the children realize how good their problem-solving ability is? The problem-solving skills of children, she believes, can be cultivated and supported and can be used to solve myriad problems, ranging from movement problems, associated with handwriting, to riding a bicycle, to organizing their desk, and so on. She is very keen on disentangling difficulties and the manner in which children try to approach activities. The essence is how children learn skills, noting that most children learn some skills essentially on their own but not all and, at times, as is the case in children with DCD, often not enough. Thus, the child could be good at soccer but not at bicycle riding. This observation agrees with the literature on the specificity of skill learning.

Helene has made a substantial contribution to the field in many ways and most individuals link her with the CO-OP. This uses a cognitive problem-solving based approach with a good evidentiary support and high uptake among clinicians and others. An essential component of the CO-OP approach is that the child is actively engaged throughout the process. The approach has seven key features:

- Client chosen goals

- Dynamic performance analysis

- Cognitive strategy use

- Guided discovery

- Enabling principles

- Parent/significant other involvement

- Intervention structure.

The emphasis is on planning and cognitive strategy use and a self-efficacy shift from 'I can't' to 'I can'. The approach includes specific guidelines on how to support the skill learning and how to actively engage the child in the process. It stresses the importance of being very specific, not general, if learning is to occur (i.e. saying 'Try harder' is of little value in the learning process). Her views on practice very much coincide with ours: we don't say 'practice makes perfect' but 'appropriate practice helps skill learning'. Helene makes the same point, warning that 'poor practice can make error perfect'!

### Dr Mellissa Prunty

Mellissa Prunty is an occupational therapist who works at Brunel University, London. As well as her academic career, Mellissa is a top-class basketball player representing her country in that sport. She has given several presentations at conferences and sees children in clinical and research settings on a regular basis. She is involved in the training of both occupational therapy and physiotherapy students and engages students in her work both research and clinical. She recently organized and hosted DCD UK 2018 conference at her University.

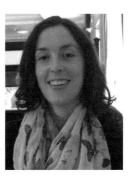

Her progression towards intervention involves the following. She recruits participants with movement disorders from ages 5 to 17 years from schools, engaging the young people and the parents in the whole research process involving both handwriting and the total movement process.

Parents often get in touch with her and she involves them in the process, taking case histories on how the children have developed, day-to-day difficulties, performance at school and their overall history and current functioning.

After taking a qualitative history, she gives the parents the MABC Checklist to complete and follows this by the MABC Test and the DASH, if appropriate.

She uses the Strengths and Difficulties Questionnaire (SDQ) to look at co-occurring difficulties, such as attention problems for handwriting in particular. She also uses the British Picture Vocabulary Scale (BVPS) for receptive language and when using the DASH she modifies it for ages below 9 years by looking at how they write the alphabet and letter formation using a digitizing writing tablet.

At the early stage of writing (age 5-6y) she focuses on letter formation and may consider aspects of grip. She reinforces correct letter formation with parents and encourages activities such as colouring. She has recently been looking at the range of movement in the joints of the hand and studying whether hypermobility plays a role in handwriting difficulties.

Whether she teaches cursive or print, writing is guided by the teacher assessment framework (Teacher assessment frameworks at the end of key stage 2, 2018), which notes that by year 6 in primary school, the children should be able to do cursive writing. She does teach print at the very beginning of the process as she feels it is easier to learn to join-up letters when the letter forms are in place.

She also engages in teaching gross motor skills such as bicycle riding. Her students are always keen to be involved in gaining experience in teaching children to do this and there is no shortage of volunteers.

She has a sports camp that includes bicycle riding and is run for 2 hours over four mornings during school holidays. The tuition is one to one, if possible, allowing for a concentration of effort from the child and the trainer. She uses task analysis for this, as she does in other skills such as tying shoe-laces, ties and ball sports.

She teaches only those activities that are chosen as goals by the children. She works with children who are diagnosed as DCD as well as those with ASD and ADHD.

### Professor Bouwien Smits-Engelsman

Bouwien Smits-Engelsman holds the position as Professor in Developmental Human movement Science at the University of Cape Town. She is a qualified physical therapist, a neuroscientist, a skilled clinician and is a prolific publisher in the area of motor rehabilitation. Bouwien is developer and co-author of the approached entitled Neuromotor Task Training (NTT), which is discussed here. NTT is a very popular, task-based approach to intervention, based upon motor learning principles and has strong support from numerous meta-analyses and systematic reviews. Bouwien gives numerous international presentations and workshops and is in constant demand for her various skills.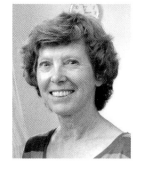

(The following description of NTT was sent directly to me by Bouwien. It is presented with one or two additions).

## Overview of the Neuromotor Task Training process

*Collecting information and planning*
**Step 1:** Start with the subjective assessment and problem identification of need. Collaborating with the child, parents and teachers to identify the tasks that the child has difficulty performing and would like to improve. These are tasks that are all from the daily functioning of the child.

**Step 2:** Selecting the tasks that the child, parents and teachers would like to work on in therapy. This is seen as a crucial step with empowerment being a basic principle and which is heightened by their choice of outcome.

**Step 3:** For each selected task, there is a systematic approach to identifying the factors that limit and enable task performance (task constraints) in different contexts. This is a skilled operation and involves careful and experienced observation of the child performing *in context*.

*Intervention*
**Step 4:** The child attends regular therapy sessions where opportunities exist to practice the task at increasing levels of difficulty and complexity, in a task-relevant environment that optimally supports learning. As the child's ability improves, tasks are progressed by increasing task difficulty and complexity. Also, transfer to school, home and leisure environment is attended to.

Although the main focus of NTT is on implicit learning and has an external focus it is also important to instruct to help the children to learn. NTT teaching involves a taxonomy of principles with the three categories of:

- **Giving instructions**: explaining, demonstrating, giving clues. The first part of learning a task is crucial: deciding which variables to pay attention to and ensuring that instructions match demonstrations.

- **Sharing knowledge**: talking about the task, asking questions and providing rhythm or timing. This is a cognitive part of skill learning.

- **Providing feedback**: what is right; what is wrong; positive and negative aspects and differentiating how these are given to children at different ages and stages in their learning and development.

### Dr Marina M Schoemaker

Marina Schoemaker is Associate Professor at the Centre of Human Movement Science, University Medical Centre Groningen, the Netherlands. Her research interests are assessment (development and evaluation of measuring instruments) and the effectiveness of intervention of children with DCD, physical fitness of children with DCD, as well as experimental studies concerning motor control mechanisms involved in upper extremity performance of children with DCD. She is a co-author of the Neuromotor Task Training along with Bouwien Smits-Engelsman. She travels world-wide giving lectures and workshops on assessment and intervention for children with movement difficulties.

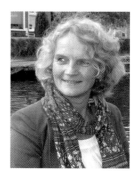

The children involved in her research come through parents who are seeking help at an outpatient rehabilitation clinic after noticing difficulties in their children. She advocates an eclectic, task-oriented approach to intervention, with NTT being an obvious approach, in combination with the work from CO-OP (see the section about Helene Polatajko), which is a cognitive motor-based approach.

Marina's emphasis is to involve parents all of the time, with some work being carried out in school and some in clinical situations. She is of the opinion that skills are given to teachers who see the child on a daily basis and thus, it is important to educate them on the basic principles of support and intervention. NTT (outlined in the Smits-Engelsman interview) provides the basis of her work, with particular emphasis of time on task. It is a well-established motor learning principle that the amount of appropriate practice is the major influencing variable in skill learning. This is the reason why Marina is keen for teachers and parents to be involved as it heightens time on task, and functional tasks can be taught. Currently, she is involved in research in which the effectiveness of a programme to increase physical fitness in children with DCD is evaluated. The programme consists of a training aspect, in which children perform exercises to increase their endurance and strength supervised by a physical therapist, and a lifestyle part, in which both parents and children are involved to encourage a more active lifestyle at home.

### Professor Peter Wilson

Peter Wilson is a developmental psychologist and movement scientist with nearly 25 years research experience. He joined the Australian Catholic University in 2012 as the Head of School of Psychology, and is currently Co-Director of the Centre for Disability and Development Research (CeDDR). He has a distinguished research background, coordinating research programmes in the field of motor and cognitive development in children, and leading research programmes on the use of

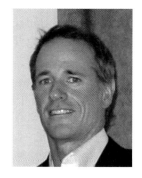

virtual-reality technology in motor and cognitive rehabilitation in adults and children. His work is strongly cross-discipline: as lead investigator on the Australian Research Council (ARC) Linkage projects, he works closely with scientists and clinicians, and collaborates extensively with colleagues internationally.

He takes a hybrid approach to research and practice (https://www.ncbi.nlm.nih.gov/pubmed/28222902), integrating cognitive neuroscience and ecological theory; taking note of the triad of variables that influence outcomes, namely the child, the task and the environment.

His work encourages careful history taking of the child together with assessment, looking at the baseline data of each child in relation to their movement goals and the performance of their typically developing peers.

His methods and techniques are informed strongly by basic research on motor control and learning. His expertise in cognitive neuroscience and developmental psychology is coupled with his initial work in physical education.

When working with the triad of influences of task-child-environment he uses the phrase 'scaling up' the task challenges, which indicates a constant monitoring and changing of task variables as the child improves.

He is a strong believer in using good and well-established motor learning principles, such as scaffolding, external focus of attention, augmented feedback and variable scheduling, to facilitate a child's progression. He believes in building up and withdrawing learning supports, and that helping the child to sense the 'feel' and 'image' of a movement is critical.

He also uses modelling, part-whole learning techniques, and may guide the child physically through a more difficult movement and then withdraw that physical support. He combines all of the above with the use of videos both for the child to watch others and to watch themselves on various tasks.

Peter is very aware that movement problems are rarely seen without associated cognitive, learning and behavioural issues, and as such, the intervention often has to accommodate these before and during the motor training.

Again, using good motor learning principles, he is a strong advocate of the importance of high intensity training, time on task, bouts of fun, and creating lots of opportunities for practice. Peter dedicates these comments to his great friend and mentor, Prof. David Sugden.

# References

Barnett A, Henderson S, Scheib B, Scholz J (2007) Detailed Assessment of Speed of Handwriting (DASH). London: Pearson.

Blank R, Barnett AL, Cairney J, et al. (2019) International clinical practice recommendations on the definition, diagnosis, assessment, intervention, and psychosocial aspects of developmental coordination disorder. *Dev Med Child Neurol* 61: 242–285.

Bronfenbrenner, U (1979) The Ecology of Human Development. Cambridge MA: Harvard Univ Press.

Doderer L, Miyahara M (2013) Critical triangulation of a movement test, questionnaires, and observational assessment for children with DCD. *International Journal of Therapy and Rehabilitation*, 20: 435–442.

Keogh JF, Sugden DA (1985) *Movement Skill Development*. New York: MacMillan.

Henderson SE, Sugden DA, Barnett A (2007) *Movement Assessment Battery for Children 2*: Kit and Manual. London: Harcourt Assessment.

Mandich AD, Polatajko HJ, Rodger S (2003) Rites of passage: understanding participation of children with developmental coordination disorder. *Hum Mov Sci* 22: 583–595.

McCarron (1976) *MAND: McCarron Assessment of Neuromuscular Development, Fine and Gross Motor Abilities* Dallas, Texas: Common Market Press.

Miyahara M, Kitada R, Sasaki A, Okamoto Y, Tanabe HC, Sadato N (2013) From gestures to words: Spontaneous verbal labeling of complex sequential hand movements reduces fMRI activation of the imitation-related regions. *Neurosci Res* 75: 228–238.

Miyahara M, Lagisz M, Nakagawa S, Henderson SE (2016) A narrative meta-review of a series of systematic and meta-analysis reviews on intervention outcomes for children with developmental coordination disorder. *Child Care Health Dev* 43: 733–742.

Miyahara M, Hillier SL, Pridham L, Nakagawa, S (2017) Task-oriented interventions for children with developmental co-ordination disorder (Review). *Cochrane Database of Systematic Reviews*. No. 7. doi/10.1002/14651858.CD010914.pub2.

Newell KM (1986) Development of coordination. In: Wade MG, Whiting HTA (eds). *Motor Development in Children: Aspects of Coordination and Control* Dordrecht. Martinus Nijhoff, pp. 341–360.

Pless M, Carlsson M (2000) Effects of motor skill intervention on developmental coordination disorder: a meta-analysis. *Adapt Phys Activ Q* 17: 381–401.

Polatajko HJ, Townsend EA, Craik J (2007) Canadian Model of Occupational Performance and Engagement (CMOP-E). In Enabling Occupation II: Advancing an Occupational Therapy Vision of Health, Well-being, & Justice through Occupation. Townsend EA & Polatajko HJ Eds. Ottawa, ON: CAOT Publications ACE. 22–36.

Preston N, Magallon S, Hill LBJ, Andrews E, Ahern SA, Mon-Williams M (2016) A systematic review of high quality randomized controlled trials investigating motor skill programmes for children with developmental coordination disorder. *Clin Rehab* 31: 857–870.

Smits-Engelsman BCM, Blank R, Van der Kaay A-C, Mosterd-Van der Meijs R, Polatajko HJ, Wilson PH (2013) Efficacy of interventions to improve motor performance in children with developmental coordination disorder: a combined systematic review and meta-analysis. *Dev Med Child Neurol* 55: 229–237.

Smits-Engelsman B, Vinçon S, Blank R, Quadrado VH, Polatajko H, Wilson PH (2018) Evaluating the evidence for motor-based interventions in developmental coordination disorder: A systematic review and meta-analysis. *Res Dev Disabil* 74: 72–102

Sugden DA, Henderson SE (2007) *Ecological Intervention for Children with Movement Difficulties.* London: Pearson.

Sugden DA, Wade MG (2013) *Typical and Atypical Motor Development.* Clinics in Developmental Medicine. London: Mac Keith Press.

Teacher assessment frameworks at the end of key stage 2 (2018) Standards and Testing Agency. ISBN 978-1-78957-211-7, STA/19/8302/e. Available at: https://www.gov.uk/government/publications/teacher-assessment-frameworks-at-the-end-of-key-stage-2 [Accessed 30 May 2019].

Wilson B, Kaplan BJ, Crawford SG, Roberts G (2007) *The Developmental Coordination Disorder Questionnaire 2007*. Calgary, Canada: Alberta Children's Hospital Decision Support Research Team.

Wilson P, Smits-Engelsman, BCM, Caeyenberghs, K & Steenbergen, B (2017) Toward a hybrid model of Developmental Coordination Disorder. Current Developmental Disorders Reports, 4, 64–71.

# Chapter 9

## At a glance: Moving forward in the right direction

### Aims and principles

The overall aim of the text is to offer guidelines and support to parents, teachers, occupational therapist and physiotherapists and other interested parties, who assist individuals showing movement difficulties. The individuals we are addressing may present movement difficulties as a primary core characteristic or may show difficulties within the context of another developmental disorder. They may or may not have a specific diagnostic condition but they will present movement difficulties in everyday activities that will interfere with general activities of daily living.

To be competent in movement based activities, two objectives stand out. The first is to be able to perform a **collection of specific functional movement skills** within an appropriate environmental context. The second is to be able to **flexibly create responses to novel movement situations across a range of environmental contexts**. The first objective requires a certain **consistency of response**, while the second requires **flexibility of movement responses, through generalization or transfer**.

Movement outcomes are a result of the transactional effect of the three variables of **child resources, environmental context** and **task selection and presentation**.

**Presentation.** The solution to movement difficulties lies within a consideration of all of these three variables as the unit of analysis, not solely the child. It is an **optimistic approach,** with many of the variables, such as environmental context, task choice, and manner of presentation, within our control.

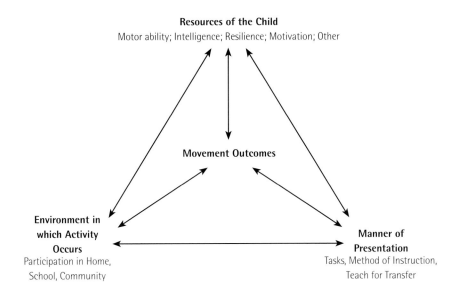

It is an **ecological model,** with different persons playing differing roles in a variety of contexts that will change over time as the individual develops and learns.

These variables are targeted to bring about an **accumulation of small gains** generating large improvement overall.

There is recognition that every child is a unique individual with specific needs requiring tailored support.

## Evidence for guidelines

Evidence is one key to effective management, support and help for any movement difficulty and can arise from three sources: **theory; empiricism; practice. Theoretical evidence** refers to the underlying principles of any intervention; **empirical evidence** is provided by experimentation as shown in randomized controlled trials, meta-analyses and reviews. **Practical evidence** is derived from professionals such as in health and/ or education, parents and families, the child and friends and other adults. These three sources of evidence often do not articulate smoothly with each other.

## Progress to intervention

Someone has raised concerns about the movement competence of an individual. It could be the individual concerned, a parent, caregiver, teacher, health professional or other. This is the initial identification.

A key worker is then required to coordinate the following activities:

- A decision is taken that the concerns are sufficient to address the difficulties through assessment and/or diagnosis leading to some form of support and intervention.

- If **DCD** is suspected, whether or not the individual is formally diagnosed, the functional symptoms are addressed. Everyday optimal functioning is the aim.

- If there is a **diagnosis of another developmental disorder** such as dyslexia, ADHD, ASD, or DLD, the movement difficulties described may show enough characteristics for an additional diagnosis of DCD to be given.

### Collecting information

There is a preference to call this stage '**collecting information**' as opposed to '**assessment**' as information on both the individual and the environmental context need to be collected. This information is derived from a **variety of sources**:

- The individual concerned

- Appropriate individual normative tests

- Appropriate criterion referenced tests

- Developmental history

- Parental interviews and reports

- Educational reports

- Health reports, including dynamic assessments

- The availability of support from family, friends, school and other educational support such as educational psychologists, health authorities.

- National, regional and local policies and practices providing assistance

- Environmental opportunities and reports within the local community.

The environmental opportunities provide a responsible person with information on whether to diagnose or not. It is recognized that in some countries a diagnosis is *required for support, which brings funding, recognition and explanation.* Care should be taken that health professionals and clinicians involved do not to have lower expectations or fulfil self-prophesies. Even without a diagnosis, the individual should receive support.

## Objectives and priorities

**Objectives**. These are **developed via multiple inputs from the different persons and perspectives. Views of the individual concerned should be a priority if at all possible**. Personally, we are all more likely to participate if all involved participate in the outcome decision.

It is better to have limited, short-term achievable objectives leading to future medium and longer-term goals.

**Priorities** can be assigned according to the following:

**Immediate need (e.g. severe disruption or self-harm)**

**Quick wins – tasks that are almost successful**

**Those that lead to other objectives (e.g. attention)**

**Enjoyment for motivation**

**Medium and longer-term goals**

## Intervention

- General guidelines

  **Scheduling**: traditional motor learning studies show that for motivational purposes little and often is preferred for practice sessions. For example, five 20-minute sessions a week is better than one 90-minute session. This is task dependent and also depends on whether short-term performance or longer -term learning is the desired outcome.

  - In addition to the more **formal practice session**s, as far as possible support should be built into **the fabric of daily life** and not always be seen as special event. If it is part of an accepted routine, the work becomes much easier. We have called this **informal practice.**
  - Health and education teams working together is always of huge benefit and the work of the CanChild in Canada (Partnering4Change) is a strong example of this.
  - As far as possible any support and practices from professionals should be cascaded to others, such as parents who daily see the individual for long periods of time. In this way, support is built into daily life and not always seen as a 'special' session.
  - A strong suggestion would be to **accumulate small gains** by involving different persons as support systems, in different areas, utilizing different contexts.

# Planning and implementing the programme involves participation and learning

*Participation*

| The child needs to find it easy to be involved | The context needs to be appropriate to child's needs | Context has to have meaning in child's life |
|---|---|---|
| **Accessibility** | **Appropriateness** | **Meaningfulness** |

- The amount of **appropriate practice** is an essential variable; it must be appropriate because inappropriate practice leads to the 'welding' in of errors.

- It assures **time on task**, a well-known known factor in the learning of many motoric skills.

- Participation needs to be **accessible appropriate and meaningful**

  - In the environmental context it calls for adjustments from **Home; School, Health and Community.**

*Learning*

- A mixture of relatively infrequent (once a week) **formal** sessions from professionals cascading practices to those in daily and long contact with individuals (parents and teachers). These more **'informal'** sessions should be built into the normal fabric of daily life.

  - Sessions – 'little and often'.

  - Work on **functional skills** not so much on form.

  - **Variability of practice** within classes of event.

  - **Different instructions**, demonstrations and feedback according to **phases of learning** individual is situated.

  - At first one to two major points, later progressing through tips to show better function, and gradually moving to dual task as the skill becomes automatic.

  - Recognize that **learning and development are non-linear** and so expect fast and slow learning with plateaus and occasionally dips.

  - Looking for **flexibility (variability) of responses** as well as consistency depending on the demands of environmental context.

- Appropriate use of **problem solving strategies.**

- Use of **expert scaffolding.**

- All practices to be **meaningful and enjoyable.**

- Use of activities that aid both **learning to move** and **moving to learn.**

- Every child is a unique individual and should receive bespoke intervention tailored to need, but not necessarily taught individually.

- With professionals, **work in groups** is always desirable aiding social context and real life experiences.

- Work for **small, marginal, achievable gains in a number of areas.**


ENGINEER THE ENVIRONMENT FOR PARTICIPATION AND DELIVER GOOD
TEACHING AND THERAPY EXPERIENCES FROM A WIDE EVIDENCE BASE.

# Index

NOTES: References to figures, boxes and tables are designated by a lower case, italic *f*, *b* and *t* respectively. "Developmental Coordination Disorder" and "Attention Deficit Hyperactivity Disorder" are abbreviated to "DCD" and "ADHD" in subheadings throughout.